Applied equine nutrition and training

Applied equine nutrition and training

Equine NUtrition and TRAining COnference (ENUTRACO) 2013

edited by: Arno Lindner

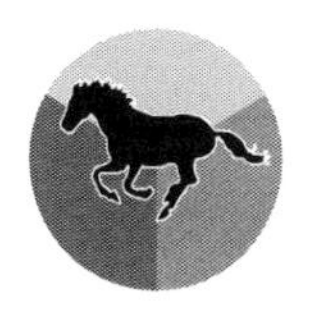

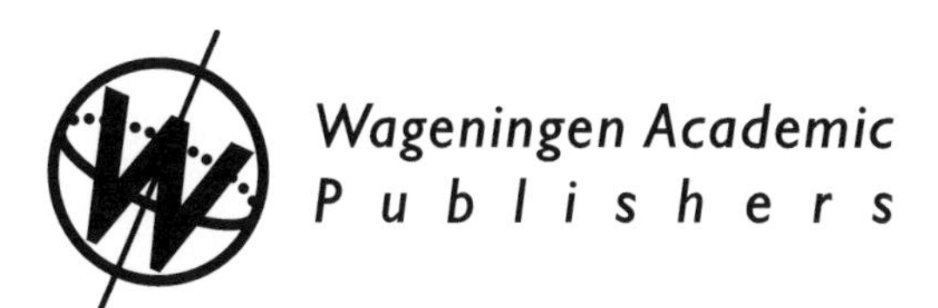

ISBN: 978-90-8686-240-5
e-ISBN: 978-90-8686-793-6
DOI: 10.3920/978-90-8686-793-6

First published, 2013

Wageningen Academic Publishers
P.O. Box 220
6700 AE Wageningen
the Netherlands
www.WageningenAcademic.com
copyright@WageningenAcademic.com

Table of contents

Expanded abstracts

Editorial

Again I am very glad and proud to present you the book of the Equine NUtrition and TRAining COnference – ENUTRACO – held in Bonn, Germany in 2013!

In this conference we decided to discuss the available information on the nutrition and training of the musculoskeletal system and to focus especially on tendons, a tissue that is frequently injured in sport horses. However, we soon realized that the musculoskeletal system would not be sufficiently covered through only nutrition and training themes, but their rehabilitation needed to be addressed too. To ensure more depth of the information we additionally have invited experts on training and rehabilitation of tendons in man. The 'product' of all efforts is here for your review! Please comment!

I owe gratitude to all involved for the insight they are giving us with their manuscripts and I wish that all readers can use these insights to keep sport horses sound and recover them better from injury!

Arno Lindner

Articles

Nutrition and the musculoskeletal system: performance vs. welfare?

Pat Harris
Mars Horsecare UK Ltd., Equine Studies Group, WALTHAM Centre for pet nutrition, Freeby lane, Waltham-on-the-Wolds LE14 4RT, United Kingdom; pat.harris@effem.com

In the wild, the horse would spend most of the day roaming and foraging in an externally variable environment as part of a herd. As non-ruminant herbivores they are well suited to a high fibre, low starch diet, would rarely fast voluntarily for more than 2-4 hours at a time and would naturally forage for 16-18 hours a day. Whilst they might roam over many kilometres each day, fast or high intensity exercise tends to be predominantly part of their 'fear and flight' response and therefore they naturally do not gallop for long distances on several occasions within a day/every day. However, domestication and our increasing demand for horses to perform at high intensities for long periods of time or repeatedly means that they may require energy intakes above those able to be provided by their more 'natural' diet of predominantly fresh forage. Whilst their digestive system as well as their 'psychology' evolved to 'cope' with a particular range of diets and life style, today most horses in the developed world are not kept as their ancestors would have lived. Modern horse management for example often brings the horse into a small-enclosed, isolated environment, limits the feeding occasions and provides large meals of cereal-based dry feeds. What and when horses are able to eat is now predominantly determined by ourselves and we therefore have to take responsibility for the effects that our choice of management practices have on their health and welfare. Unfortunately some of our choices may not be optimal for equine welfare (Davidson and Harris, 2002).

This is therefore the primary challenge – how do we provide sufficient energy and other nutrients to fuel and support optimal muscular-skeletal functioning whilst minimising any associated risks to health and welfare. Animal welfare can be defined ecologically as the good fit of an animal to its environment, which can be evaluated from the point of view of the animal and its adaptation, or alternatively from how the environment can be adapted to the animal, for example, by improved housing, training or feeding. This paper will explore some of the dilemmas facing owners and feeders of horses who want to maximise the athletic capability of their horse but ideally minimise any compromise to their welfare. It will concentrate on energy and protein provision as these are perhaps the areas where potential conflicts between welfare and performance are the most obvious.

What about energy provision?

We all recognise that without sufficient energy a horse cannot grow or perform regardless of the breed or discipline involved. Energy is supplied to the horse via its diet, but fundamentally energy is not a nutrient. The chemical energy or gross energy contained within feeds is converted into net or useable energy. Different feeds and feedstuffs contain differing amount of the raw chemical energy and the efficiency of their conversion to useable or net energy also differs widely. Cereals have more net energy than hay does; hay contains more than twice the net or useable energy than straw (Ellis, 2013). The first performance enhancing aid in fact may have been barley which was found in Ancient Grecian times to support performance by providing additional energy over and above forage. Cereals have been commonly fed to horses ever since, primarily as a concentrated energy source due to their high starch content. Horses have a finite capacity/appetite and therefore energy dense feeds are potentially very valuable. So why is there so much concern today? It is because on one hand we increasingly realise that high starch and sugar diets increase the risk of gastrointestinal problems (including gastric ulcers and some types of colic; Durham, 2013; Luthersson and Nadeau, 2013), behaviour issues (Hothersall and Nicol, 2013) and in certain animals the risk of muscular problems (Harris and Rivero, 2013) as well as laminitis (Geor and Harris, 2013). But on the other hand there are concerns that high performance horses (1) cannot eat sufficient forage to support optimal performance; (2) forage only diets will reduce performance due to 'gut fill'; and (3) adversely affect muscle glycogen content. These aspects will be explored in more detail below.

Issue over muscle glycogen content and replenishment

The chemical energy or gross energy contained within feeds is converted ultimately into adenosine triphosphate (ATP). Muscles only have a small store of ATP – only enough for 1-2 seconds of exercise. Creatine phosphate stores may help support ATP production and utilisation for a few more seconds – but then the muscles have to re-synthesise ATP (Geor, 2013; Harris, 1997). Stored energy, primarily in the form of muscle and liver glycogen as well as intramuscular and adipose triglycerides, are used to provide this ATP. Short-term, intense exercise and longer duration, submaximal exercise can significantly affect muscle glycogen stores and low muscle glycogen content can contribute to skeletal muscle fatigue and poor performance (Harris *et al.*, 1987; Hodgson *et al.*, 1984; Lacombe *et al.*, 2001; Snow *et al.*, 1987; Topliff *et al.*, 1983). Glycogen loss during normal race-like training may be accommodated easily by a normal diet containing concentrates or even just good quality forage (Snow and Harris, 1991) and is unlikely to lead to depletion prior to racing unless repeated intensive work is undertaken with insufficient time between the bouts – which does occur with certain training programmes. Insufficient recovery time may also be an issue with multi-day events or where multiple competitions occur on the same day/day after day, i.e. for eventers/ show jumpers, multiple day endurance rides, etc.

Diets that support high basal muscle glycogen content as well as good restoration post exercise theoretically then should be a potential goal of the feeding strategy for performance horses. For us humans, it appears that a diet high in starch and sugar is optimal for restoration of muscle glycogen stores, and diet also can be manipulated to increase basal glycogen content. The normal glycogen content of rested human muscle is approximately 300 mmol/kg dry matter (dm), but may be increased 2-fold by a combination of exercise and diet. The use of 'glycogen loading' stems from early work in man (Bergström *et al.*, 1967) and previously it involved a 3-4 day depletion phase of hard training on a low carbohydrate diet followed by a 3-4 day loading phase of high carbohydrate intake with tapering of the exercise. However, today it more commonly tends to involve 3 days of tapering exercise combined with a high carbohydrate intake ~7-10 g/kg body weight (BW)/day (Burke, 2000). Muscle glycogen synthetic rates of 5-8 mmol/kg/h can be achieved in man with the intake of carbohydrate at a rate of 0.7-1.0 g/kg BW every 2 h during the 6-12 h period after glycogen-depleting exercise with complete glycogen replenishment occurring within 24 hours (Burke, 2000).

However, it appears to be very difficult to improve the rate of glycogen recovery in the horse *safely* nutritionally (Harris *et al.*, 2013). The 'safely' is a key point given that approximately 7-10 kg of oats would be required to be fed to a 500 kg horse to approximate to the daily dose fed to human athletes to result in glycogen loading (7-10 g/kg BW/day). Whilst some horses might eat this amount when in race training:

- No beneficial effect on performance has been shown in horses with very high sugar and starch diets (Essen-Gustavsson *et al.*, 1991; Poso *et al.*, 2005).
- Some epidemiological studies have identified the level of grain feeding as a risk factor for colic (Durham, 2013), e.g. odds ratios of 4.8 and 6.3 (relative to no episode of colic) have been reported for horses fed, respectively, 2.5 kg/day and more than 5.0 kg/day of concentrate (Tinker *et al.*, 1997).
- Similarly, recent (within the previous 2 weeks) changes in the type or amount of grain or concentrate fed, or feeding more than 2.7 kg of oats per day have been associated with increased risk for an episode of colic (Hudson *et al.*, 2001).
- High cereal based diets by necessity (due to appetite limitations) tend to be linked with low fibre/forage based diets which may predispose horses to behavioural issues as well as gastrointestinal dysfunction (e.g. gastric ulcers, colic; Durham, 2013; Luthersson and Nadeau, 2013).

Standardbred horses in training, fed a forage:concentrate diet with a starch intake of 0.54 g/kg BW per day, showed a reduced microbial stability and an increase in the faecal flora of lactic acid bacteria and members of the *Streptococcus bovis/equis* complex when compared to the feeding of a forage-only diet (Willing *et al.*, 2009).

And the question would still be whether such high and regular intakes of starch and sugar would even result in an improved rate of glycogen restoration. To date in horses, the maximum rate of muscle glycogen synthesis that has been reported is approximately 1-2 mmol/kg/h with oral feeding and complete recovery taking as long as 48-72 h (Hyppa *et al.*, 1997; Lacombe *et al.*, 2004; Snow *et al.*, 1987). The type of diet fed appears to makes little difference over this period of time as illustrated by one study where glycogen repletion, following exercise that resulted in a 40% decrease in the muscle store, was approximately the same in horses fed a low carbohydrate (LC) diet consisting of hay, a normal carbohydrate (NC) diet consisting of pelleted concentrate plus hay, or a high carbohydrate (HC) diet, which was the NC diet supplemented with i.v. infusions of 0.45 kg glucose (~0.9 g/kg BW) on each of the first 2 days (Snow *et al.*, 1987). An increased rate of glycogen re-synthesis was observed by Davie *et al.* (1995), however, when 6 g/kg BW dextrose was infused i.v. following exercise (which resulted in a 50%, decrease in the muscle content). However, it seems that any advantage gained in the repletion of the muscle glycogen stores, even by this or other rather extreme procedures is short-lived (Cunilleras *et al.*, 2006) and the high starch (cereal grain) feeding regimens used in various studies has only resulted if anything in a modest gain in glycogen synthesis rate (Cunilleras *et al.*, 2006; Geor, 2013; Lacombe *et al.*, 2004). Some work suggests that the source and availability of sugars in the diet may affect glycogen utilization and possibly performance, e.g. muscle glycogen utilisation was lowered on diets with high sugar content (barley syrup content compared to diets with oats; Jansson *et al.*, 2002) – but further work is needed before clear advice on this aspect can be given. Other nutritional treatments that have been shown to enhance glycogen restoration in man also do not appear to affect glycogen synthesis rate in horses. However recently it has been suggested that the restoration of hydration and electrolyte/acid-base balance may be more important to the enhancement of glycogen synthesis than additional glucose load (Waller *et al.*, 2009; Waller and Lindinger, 2010).

What about oil then?

Glycogen-sparing is one of the most commonly considered ergogenic effects of oil inclusion which could lead to delayed fatigue and improved performance especially in endurance activities (Griewe *et al.*, 1989; Harris, 1997; Pagan *et al.*, 1987, 2002). The effect on high intensity exercise capacity is perhaps more controversial with some, but not all research, showing *potential* for improved high intensity exercise performance. Any potential improvement might be due to increased energy production via anaerobic glycolysis because of either higher muscle glycogen stores and/or altered regulation of glycogenolysis (Harris, 1997; Kronfeld *et al.*, 1998). However, the effect of oil supplementation on basal glycogen content is itself controversial (Geor, 2013; Waller and Lindinger, 2010) with some reporting an increase, some no effect and others even a decrease! In addition, evidence that adaptation to oil supplementation affects performance *per se* in the field (above and beyond potential positive effects on behaviour, thermal load, energy provision, reduction in starch intake, etc.) is still required.

The amount of oil that should be added (with respect to energy provision) is also still open to some debate. Horses have been shown to be able to digest and utilise up to 20% or more of the diet as oil. A relationship between dietary fat and muscle glycogen concentration has apparently indicated a peak glycogen at 12% oil by weight. A number of trials have suggested possible benefits of incorporating this much oil in a complete and balanced feed (Kronfeld and Harris, 1997). However, some studies have suggested very high intakes of oil may reduce muscle glycogen concentrations, which as mentioned above is not desirable. Adding oil to existing feed also has the potential to create multiple imbalances and therefore could be considered less safe than feeding a diet where the oil has been balanced in relation to all of the essential nutrients in the feed. Levels of 5-8% in the total diet are therefore more commonly recommended as the typical upper limit and as an initial guide (without specific nutritional advice) up to 1 ml/kg BW/day can be fed. Certainly, the majority of animals (500 kg BW) can be supplemented up to 400 mls/day (~370 g) in divided doses – provided that the oil has been introduced gradually, *is required* and is not rancid (and the vitamin E levels are considered: see below). In order to obtain any possible metabolic benefits from the feeding of oil, in addition to those associated with its high energy density and lack of starch content, the oil probably needs to be fed for several weeks/months (Harris, 1997; Kronfeld and Harris, 1997; Pagan *et al.*, 2002).

It is, however, very important to note that oil does not provide any additional protein, vitamins (vitamin E content is variable) or minerals. If the horse is not receiving sufficient of these nutrients, for its workload, from its basal diet, then an appropriate additional vitamin and mineral mix may be needed and it is recommended that additional Vitamin E be fed in combination with supplemental oil. Exact recommendations are not known but an additional 1-1.5 iu

Vitamin E per ml added supplemental oil has been suggested (Harris and Arkell, 2005; Zeyner and Harris, 2013).

Why not just feed forage and arrange training/performance times around the optimal restoration rates?

Whilst it might be possible to allow at least 72 hours between competitions, for some this would not be possible like the 3 day eventer or showjumper. And what about effects of forage only diets on performance – recently there have been a number of studies from Sweden looking into the possibility to train and compete Standardbred racehorses on high energy (ie immature early cut) forage only diets (Connysson *et al.*, 2006; 2010; Jansson and Lindberg, 2012; Muhonen *et al.*, 2009). They have shown that horses in training can maintain body-condition and BW on forage only diets and have suggested that the effects on metabolic responses to exercise potentially could be beneficial. One key issue, however, relates back to glycogen as this work suggests that the muscle glycogen contents of forage only fed Standardbred trotters in exercise training can be lower (~13%; Jansson and Lindberg, 2012) than those reported for horses maintained on conventional forage/grain rations. In an earlier reported study similar glycogen contents were found (Essén-Gustavsson *et al.*, 2010) when fed a higher protein providing forage, however, this forage was also higher in its water soluble carbohydrate (WSC) content and therefore currently it is not known whether the effect on muscle glycogen content was due to the higher CP, WSC, or some other factor. Nevertheless this is interesting work that needs to be continued. Ideally it should also be undertaken in other types of performance horses in particular thoroughbred racehorses as anecdotally, they appear to perform better when the ration contains some starch (and simple sugar), with the currently unsubstantiated suggestion that muscle glycogen concentrations are suboptimal when the diet provides <10% DE from starch and simple sugar.

Other potential issues include concerns over thermal load as well as appetite (and total energy intake), however, perhaps the main reason that most trainers are reluctant to feed high forage based diets is that for every kilogram of average dry hay, around 2.5-3.5 kg of water may be consumed; this will add to the weight of the horse and may adversely affect performance. Therefore, many trainers believe that forage should be restricted to reduce gut fill and therefore body weight in high performance horses. For this and other reasons the preference is to feed large amounts of high energy cereals and reduced amounts of 'bulking' forage. There certainly is some evidence that a short-term reduction in forage intake may be beneficial in horses undertaking high-intensity exercise. When compared to *ad libitum* hay consumption, restricting hay intake to ~1% of BW for a 3-day period before a treadmill exercise test (2 min at 115% VO_{2max}) resulted in a 2% decrease in body weight and a reduction in anaerobic energy expenditure during exercise, as evidenced by reduced oxygen deficit and plasma lactate concentrations. The reduction in body weight was attributed to a decrease in bowel ballast (gut fill) (Rice *et al.*, 2001). However, the practical implications of these findings are uncertain given that many racehorses do not consume more than 1% of BW of forage routinely. In fact, the actual feeding value or quality of the forage can have as much of an effect on gut fill and water turnover as the amount of forage being fed. As discussed by Harris *et al.* (2013), if we compare the feeding of 10 kg DM hay with either low (40%) or high (70%) DM digestibility these two rations will result in 6 and 3 kg of undigested DM, respectively. Assuming a consistent faecal water content (20% DM in faeces), the low and high digestibility hays will require 24 l and 12 l of water, respectively. In other words, the lower digestibility hay will result in a doubling of gut fill at the same level of intake. Therefore, high performance horses should be fed high quality forage to minimize the impact on gut fill.

In conclusion the author's current recommendations (see also Harris *et al.*, 2013) are that we should feed forage (grass and preserved forages) at 15 g DM/kg BW/day even to those animals with high energy requirements (in which case young less mature high energy providing forages should be considered). Plus the absolute minimal level for animals undergoing restriction for weight loss purposes is 10 g DM/kg BW/day (of a low energy providing forage) and a target level even in racing animals would be 12.5 g DM/kg BW/day (of a high energy providing forage). Another key point is that many hays, at least in the UK, may be low in protein (Longland *et al.*, 2013) as well as deficient in vitamins and minerals, and therefore appropriate supplementation will be required for most horses but especially performance horses on a forage rich diet.

What about protein?

During a program of physical conditioning (exercise training) there is a substantial change in protein metabolism, including increased turnover of muscle proteins and an increase in endogenous losses in association with increased feed ingestion and sweat production (Urschel and Lawrence, 2013). Dietary protein requirements of exercising horses are higher when compared to animals at maintenance, although we do not currently know the optimal intakes of protein/amino acids required to support optimal functioning/repair, etc. This can result in issues, in that feeding unnecessarily high intakes of protein will add to the thermal load of the animal as protein is inefficiently converted to useable energy, with proportionally higher amounts of waste energy (heat) produced. Oxidation of the phosphorus and sulphur in protein adds to the acid load on the body and as excess protein cannot be stored the excess nitrogen must be removed from the body, resulting in increased water requirements (the excess protein is lost primarily as urea in the urine). This leads to a potential welfare issue for stabled animals as they cannot move away from their excreta and the higher levels of urea in the urine may lead to higher environmental ammonia as the excreted urea is converted to ammonia – adding to the 'stress' on the respiratory system of stabled animals. There have been suggestions in the past that high protein intakes will negatively affect performance (e.g. Glade *et al.*, 1993) but as there were confounding factors further work is needed in this area. Certainly in other species there is some evidence that very high protein intakes may actually have a negative effect on muscle function but again the practical relevance of these results to the equine athlete is perhaps questionable given that even a very high protein diet for a horse would tend to be a low to low/moderate protein diet in other animals. Another key point is the quality (i.e. amino acid profile) of the forage and currently the author recommends that unless the quality of the protein is known most high performance horses should still be fed at least 2 g CP/kg BW/day and for those in very intense work up to 3 g CP/kg BW/day may be advisable (providing stable hygiene is good and water intake is not restricted). With respect to the key amino acids currently the author recommends around 0.08-0.1 g/kg BW/day lysine and 0.64-0.8 g threonine/kg BW/day. The amount of additional lysine needed will depend on the hay and pasture being fed and the nature of any additional energy sources.

Finally, last but not least, it is important to maintain good hydration as well as good stable hygiene and management.

So what about the skeletal system?

Here the major nutritional associated welfare issues include those of diet and management increasing the risk of developmental orthopaedic disease (DOD) of growing foals potentially through the desire to have larger more mature animals at an earlier age. The term DOD may be considered to be first coined in the 1980's to encompass all orthopaedic problems seen in the growing horse and therefore it is non-specific and the definitions are not uniformly agreed. However, in general today DOD is taken to include (Vervuert and Ellis, 2013) the following conditions: physitis, osteochondrosis (OC), acquired angular limb deformities, flexural deformities, tarsal bone collapse, cervical vertebral malformation, and acquired vertebral deformities. It has been suggested that the clinical signs of OC occur only after a progression of events that begin with a disturbance in the normal development of the cartilage (sometimes referred to as dyschondroplasia: DCP) leading to OC. At this point physical stresses are superimposed, leading to clinical signs. It is also thought possible that the initial defects/lesions may heal or develop into OC or into subchondral bone cysts. Due to the multifactorial nature of DOD, no single cause is likely to result in expression. Factors that may contribute include a genetic disposition, biomechanical trauma, and mechanical stress through inappropriate exercise, obesity, rapid growth and inappropriate or imbalanced nutrition. Different combinations may be involved in different cases. Environmental or managemental factors most likely determine if expression occurs (i.e. provide the final triggering factor(s); Harris *et al.*, 2005; Vervuert and Ellis, 2013).

What is the evidence re link between energy supply and DOD

It should be noted that there has been concern that the lesions produced by many research studies, some of which are summarised below, are not directly comparable to those found in the field (van Weeren, 2006; Vervuert and Ellis, 2013) and many field studies have reported foals being fed much higher energy intakes without an apparent increase in clinical incidence (e.g. Kronfeld, 1990). This may be linked perhaps to the background level of predisposition within the individuals, nature of the energy being provided and the balance of the diet.

- Feeding 129% NRC energy requirements to foals from 130 days of age resulted in an increased incidence of lesions compared with the control group (fed 100%) or those fed 126% of the National Research council's recommendations (NRC, 1989) for protein (Savage *et al.*, 1993). Multiple lesions of dyschondroplasia (DCP) were found on gross post mortem in 11 foals fed the high DE diet; one fed the high protein diet and one fed the control diet. Histological lesions of DCP were found in 18 foals: in all 12 of the high DE, four of the high protein and 2 of the control foals.
- Cymbaluk *et al.* (1990) reported *ad libitum* cube feeding resulted in a higher incidence of conformational and locomotor abnormalities at 25 months of age than the more restricted diet.
- Glade and Belling (1984) compared the growth of foals fed either 70 (R) or 130% (H) of the NRC (1978) recommended levels for energy. The H group showed developmental disturbances of growth plates whereas the R group had normal development of the bones but at reduced speed.
- A detailed longitudinal growth study of 18 colts split into either limited or *ad libitum* fed groups illustrated more rapid growth and a higher incidence of clinically assessed conformational and musculoskeletal abnormalities in the *ad libitum* fed group (Cymbaluk *et al.*, 1990).

In fact growth rate depends on both genetics and nutrition. Rapid growth rates and high-energy intakes have been regularly included in the list of potential multiple causes of DOD (Harris *et al.*, 2005). As discussed by these authors, the direct relationship of these causes with the various manifestations of DOD has proven elusive. The difficulty is due to the complexities that relate energy intake to growth rate and normal or abnormal skeletal development. Especially when, in order for the rapid growth rate to occur a combination of genetic ability to grow rapidly and the nutrition to support at least in part such growth is required. Energy is available to the horse in numerous forms, each of which is used with a different efficiency and have distinctive effects on hormonal systems related to growth (somatotropic axis). The relationship is further complicated by genetic differences. It is also important to note that a lack of rapid growth does not necessarily protect against an increased incidence of DOD, e.g. in the study of

Savage *et al.* (1993b) the high P diet resulted in lesions of DCP despite a trend towards a depression in average daily gain (non-significant).

So is there any recent evidence from the field linking energy/protein intakes and OC

Several studies have provided supportive evidence that the type of energy sources provided in the diet may influence certain key hormones that might in turn be involved in the pathophysiology of DOD (Harris *et al.*, 2005; Vervuert and Ellis, 2013). Previous work has, for example, linked diets/individuals which have higher glycaemic and insulinaemic responses with an increased risk of OC (Pagan *et al.*, 2001; Ralston, 2002). A fairly recent study in Germany however, apparently failed to find any apparent significant link between the feeding management of foals and the incidence of OC (Borchers, 2002; Wilke *et al.*, 2003). With respect to nutrition no relationship was found between the nutritional status of the mares (in relation to digestible crude protein and digestible energy) and the incidence of OC. However, for a number of reasons (e.g. when stabled, foals were not fed separately from the mares, estimations were used to determine milk and pasture intakes, etc.) the nutritional status of the foals could not be determined accurately (Borchers, 2002). This was also the case in a more recent study (Vander Heyden *et al.*, 2013), which looked at the feeding practices and housing management of 223 Belgian Warmblood foals using a multivariate model to determine risk factors for OC in three periods: gestation, birth to weaning and weaning to one-year-old. In this study no apparent effect of the type of feeding of the foal before or after weaning was reported, but again limited information was available to the researchers with respect to the type of feed and how much was being fed etc. This study did, however, suggest that there may be a significant relationship between OC development and: (1) the maternal nutrition during gestation; and (2) the type of housing of the foals during their first year. The authors suggested for example that mares fed with concentrates during gestation were more likely to produce foals that are subsequently affected by OC compared with other mares ($P<0.05$). However, the exact nature of these 'concentrates' is not known, although the authors comment that dietary-induced insulin resistance in pregnant mares could play a role in the aetiology of OC – suggesting perhaps that they believed the majority to be high starch/sugar based rations. More work is obviously needed in this area although whether this should be under field conditions or controlled conditions (in which the diet is known or can be accurately determined) is an interesting question.

Conclusion

There are many other obvious examples of potential welfare:muscular skeletal performance dilemmas, for example in order to reduce the risk of injury, control feed intake, etc., many high performance horses spend all or most of their time being stabled – this limits obviously their free movement and usually contact with other horses, etc. Stabling *per se* also increases the risk of lung inflammation and the feeding of, or bedding on forage, with a poor hygiene quality will increase the risk even further (Kamphues, 2013). This highlights the point that we can minimise some potential negative impacts of our managemental practices – as suggested in the introduction – in this case by providing clean bedding and forage of good hygienic quality. Therefore, it is very important when considering the care and management of our horses that we consider such aspects.

But what about the less obvious – for example muscle activity is associated with oxidative stress and the animal needs appropriate antioxidant capacity to minimise the adverse effects of the free radicals produced – are we compromising horse welfare if we fail to provide adequate antioxidant nutrition or may we compromise adaptation if we provide excessive supplementation? Similarly high performance exercise, at least in other species, can lead to adverse effects on the immune system and an increased risk of certain diseases – again are we compromising welfare of our horses if we fail to provide *optimal* nutritional support for the immune system? This leads us inevitably however to the fact that often we do not have all the answers as to how to feed our high performance horses optimally to support all the challenges that being a high performance horse imposes. But this does mean we should use all the knowledge available to us in order to try and minimise any potential adverse effects on their health and welfare whilst still supporting high performance.

References

Bergström, J., Hermansen, L., Hultman, E. and Saltin, B., 1967. Diet, muscle glycogen and physical performance. Acta Physiologica Scandinavica 71: 140-150.

Borchers, A., 2002. Die Körpergewichts- und Körpergrößenentwicklung des Warmblutfohlens während des ersten Lebenshalbjahres in Bezug zur Energie- und Proteinzufuhr sowie zum Auftreten der Osteochondrose [Bodyweight and physical development of Warmbloodfoals during the first 6 months of life in relation to energy and protein supply and occurrence of osteochondrosis]. Doctoral thesis, Veterinary University Hanover, Hanover Germany.

Burke, L., 2000. Preparation for competition. In: Clinical Sports Nutrition, Eds: L. Burke and V. Deakin, Roseville, McGraw-Hill, New York, NY, USA, pp. 341-368.

Connysson, M., Essen-Gustavsson, B., Lindberg, J.E. and Jansson, A., 2010. Effects of feed deprivation on Standardbred horses in training fed a forage-only diet and a 50:50 forage-oats diet. Equine Veterinary Journal Supplement 38: 335-340.

Connysson, M., Muhonen, S., Lindberg, J.E., Essen-Gustavsson, B., Nyman, G., Nostell, K. and Jansson, A., 2006. Effects on exercise response, fluid and acid-base balance of protein intake from forage-only diets in Standardbred horses. Equine Veterinary Journal Supplement 36: 648-653.

Cunilleras J.E., Hinchcliff, K.W., Lacombe, V.A., Sams, R.A., Kohn, C.W., Taylor, L.E. and Devor, S.T., 2006. Ingestion of starch-rich meals after exercise increases glucose kinetics but fails to enhance muscle glycogen replenishment in horses. Veterinary Journal 171: 468-477.

Cymbaluk, N.F., Christison, G.I., and Leach, D.H., 1990. Longitudinal growth analysis of horses following limited and *ad libitum* feeding. Equine Veterinary Journal 22: 198-204.

Davidson, N. and Harris, P., 2002. Nutrition and Welfare. In: Waran, N. (ed.) The welfare of horses. Kluwer Academic publishers, Dordrecht, Netherlands, pp. 45-76.

Davie, A.J., Evans, D.L., Hodgson, D.R. and Rose, R.J., 1995. Effects of intravenous dextrose infusion on muscle glycogen resynthesis after intense exercise. Equine Exercise Physiology 4. Equine Veterinary Journal Suppl. 18: 195-198.

Durham, A., 2013. Intestinal disease. In: Geor, R.J., Harris, P.A., Coenen, M. (eds.), Equine clinical and applied nutrition. Elsevier Inc, Philadelphia, PA, USA, pp. 568-581.

Ellis, A., 2013. Energy systems and requirements. In: Geor, R.J., Harris, P.A., Coenen, M. (eds.), Equine clinical and applied nutrition. Elsevier Inc, Philadelphia, PA, USA, pp. 96-112.

Essen-Gustavsson, B., Blomstrand, E., Karlstrom, K., Lindholm, A. and Persson, S.G.B., 1991. Influence of diet on substrate metabolism during exercise. In: Persson, S.G.B., Lindholm, A. and Jeffcott, L.B. (eds.), Equine Exercise Physiology 3, ICEEP Publications, Davis, CA, USA, pp. 288-298.

Essen-Gustavsson, B., Connysson, M. and Jansson, A. 2010. Effects of crude protein intake from forage-only diets on muscle amino acids and glycogen levels in horses in training. Equine Veterinary Journal 38: 341-346.

Geor, R.J., 2013. Endocrine and metabolic physiology. In: Geor, R.J., Harris, P.A., Coenen, M. (eds.), Equine clinical and applied nutrition. Elsevier Inc., Philadelphia, PA, USA, pp. 33-63.

Geor, R.J., and Harris, P.A., 2013. Laminitis. In: Geor, R.J., Harris, P.A., Coenen, M. (eds.), Equine clinical and applied nutrition. Elsevier Inc, Philadelphia, PA, USA, pp. 469-486.

Glade, M.J. and Belling, T.H., 1986. A dietary etiology for osteochondroitic cartilage. Journal of Equine Veterinary Science 6: 175-187.

Griewe, K.M., Meacham, T.N. and Fontenot, J.P., 1989. Effect of added dietary fat on exercising horses. In: Proc. 11th Equine Nutrition and Physiology symposium, Stillwater , OK, USA, pp. 101-106.

Harris, P., Staniar, W. and Ellis, A., 2005. Effect of exercise and diet on the incidence of DOD in the Growing horse: nutrition and prevention of growth disorders. In: Julliand, V. and Martin-Rosset, W. (eds.), EEAP Publication No. 114, Wageningen Academic Publishers, Wageningen, the Netherlands, pp. 273-291.

Harris, P.A. and Arkell, K., 2005. How understanding the digestive process can help minimise digestive disturbances. In: Harris, P.A., Mair, T.S., Slater, J.D. and Green, R.E. (eds.), Equine nutrition for all, Proceedings of the 1st BEVA & WALTHAM Nutrition symposia Harrogate, UK, pp. 9-14.

Harris, P.A. and Rivero, J-L.L., 2013. Exercise associated muscle disorders. In: Geor, R.J., Harris, P.A., Coenen, M. (eds.), Equine clinical and applied nutrition. Elsevier Inc, Philadelphia, PA, USA, pp. 521-535.

Harris, P.A., 1997. Energy requirements of the exercising horse. Annual review of Nutrition 17: 185-210.

Harris, P.A., Coenen, M. and Geor, R.J., 2013. Controversial areas in equine nutrition and feeding management: the editors' views. In: Geor, R.J., Harris, P.A., Coenen, M. (eds.), Equine clinical and applied nutrition. Elsevier Inc., Philadelphia, PA, USA, pp. 455-468.

Harris, R.C., Marlin, D.J. and Snow, D.H., 1987. Metabolic response to maximal exercise of 800 and 2000 m in the thoroughbred horse. Journal of Applied Physiology 63: 12-19.

Hodgson, D.R., Rose, R.J., Allen, J.R. and DiMauro, J., 1984. Glycogen depletion patters in horses performing maximal exercise. Research in Veterinary Science 36: 169-173.

Hothersall, B. and Nicol, C.J., 2013. Effects of diet on behaviour – normal and abnormal. In: Geor, R.J., Harris, P.A., Coenen, M. (eds.), Equine Clinical and Applied nutrition. Elsevier Inc, Philadelphia, PA, USA, pp. 443-454.

Hudson, J.M., Cohen, N.D., Gibbs, P.G. and Thompson, J.A., 2001. Feeding practices associated with colic in horses. Journal of American Veterinary Medical Association 219: 1419-1425.

Hyyppä, S., Rasanen, L.A. and Pösö, A.R., 1997. Resynthesis of glycogen in skeletal muscle from Standardbred trotters after repeated bouts of exercise. American Journal of veterinary Research 58: 162-166.

Jansson, A. and Lindberg, J.E., 2012. A forage only diet alters the metabolic response of horses in training. Animal 6: 1939-1946.

Jansson, A., Nyman, S., Lindholm, A. and Lindberg, J.E., 2002. Effect of exercise metabolism of varying dietary starch and sugar proportions Equine Veterinary Journal Supplement 34: 17-21.

Kamphues, J., 2013. Feed Hygiene and related disorders in horses In: Geor, R.J., Harris, P.A., Coenen, M. (eds.), Equine Clinical and Applied nutrition. Elsevier Inc, Philadelphia, PA, USA, pp 367-380.

Kronfeld, D. and Harris, P.A., 1997. Feeding the athletic horse. In: Thompson, K.N. (ed.), The veterinarians Practical reference to Equine Nutrition. American Association of Equine Practitioners, Lexington, KY, USA, pp. 61-77.

Kronfeld, D.S., 1990. Dietary aspects of Developmental Orthopedic disease in young horses Veterinary Clinics of North America: Equine Practice 6: 451-465.

Kronfeld, D.S., Custalow, S.E., Ferrante, P.L., Taylor, L.E., Wilson, J.A. and Tiegs, W., 1998. Acid-base responses of fat-adapted horses: relevance to hard work in the heat. Applied animal Behaviour 59: 61-72.

Lacombe, V., Hinchcliff, K.W., Geor, R.J. and Baskin, C.A. (2001. Muscle glycogen depletion and subsequent replenishment affect anaerobic capacity of horses. Journal of applied Physiology 91: 1782-1790.

Lacombe, V.A., Hinchcliff, K.W., Kohn, C.W., Devor, S.T. and Taylor, L.E., 2004. Effects of feeding meals with various soluble carbohydrate content on muscle glycogen synthesis after exercise in horses. American journal of veterinary Research 65: 916-923.

Longland, A., Barfoot, C. and Harris, P.A., 2013. Effect of water temperature and agitation on loss of water-soluble carbohydrates and protein from grass hay: implications for equine feeding management. Veterinary Record (in press).

Luthersson, N. and Nadeau, J.A., 2013. Gastric Ulceration. In: Geor, R.J., Harris, P.A., Coenen, M. (eds.), Equine Clinical and Applied nutrition. Elsevier Inc, Philadelphia, PA, USA, pp. 558-567.

Muhonen, S., Lindberg, J.E., Bertilsson, J. and Jansson, A., 2009. Effects on fluid balance and exercise response in Standardbred horses feed silage, haylage and hay. Comparative Exercise Physiology 5: 133-142.

NRC, 1989. Nutrient requirements of horses 5th edition. Washington DC. National Academy Press, Washington, DC, USA.

Pagan, J.D., Essen-Gustavsson, B., Lindholm, A. and Thornton J., 1987. The effect of dietary energy source on exercise performance in Standardbred horses. In: Gillespie, J.R. and Robinson, N.E. (eds.), Equine Exercise Physiology 2. ICEEP publications, Davis, CA, USA, pp. 686-700.

Pagan, J.D., Geor, R.J., Caddel, S.E., Pryor, P.B. and Hoekstra, K.E., 2001. The relationship between glycaemic response and the incidence of OCD in thoroughbred weanlings: A field study. In: Proceedings of the Annual Convention of the America Association of Equine Practitioners, Lexington, KY, USA, pp. 322-325.

Pagan, J.D., Geor, R.J., Harris, P.A., Hoekstra, K., Gardner, S., Hudson, C. and Prince, A., 2002. Effects of fat adaptation on glucose kinetics and substrate oxidation during low intensity exercise. Equine Veterinary Journal Suppl. 34: 33-39.

Poso, R.A., Hyyppa, S. and Geor, R., 2004. Metabolic responses to exercise and training. In: Hinchcliff, K.W., Kaneps, A.J., Geor, R.J. and Bayly, W. (eds.), Equine Sports Medicine and Surgery. Saunders, London, England, pp. 853-871.

Ralston, S.L., 1996. Hyperglycaemic/hyperinsulinemia after feeding a meal of grain to young horses with osteochondrosis dissecans (OCD) lesions. Pferdeheilkunde 12: 320-322.

Rice, O., Geor, R., Harris, P., Hoekstra, K., Gardner, S. and Pagan, J., 2001. Effects of restricted hay intake on body weight and metabolic responses to high intensity exercise in thoroughbred horses. Proceedings of Equine Nutrition and Physiology society, Lexington, KY, USA, pp. 273-279.

Savage, C.J., McCarthy, R.N. and Jeffcott, L.B., 1993. Effects of dietary energy and protein on induction of dyschondroplasia in foals. Equine Veterinary Journal Suppl. 16: 74-79.

Snow, D.H. and Harris, R.C., 1991. Effects of daily exercise on muscle glycogen in the thoroughbred racehorse. In: Persson, S.G.B., Lindolm, A. and Jeffcott, L.B. (eds.), Equine Exercise Physiology 3, ICEEP Publications, Davis, CA, USA, pp. 299-304.

Snow, D.H., Harris, R.C., Harman, J. and Marlin, D.J., 1987. Glycogen repletion following different diets. In: Gillespie, J.R. and Robinson, N.E. (eds.), Equine Exercise Physiology 2. ICEEP publications, Davis, CA, USA, pp. 701-710.

Tinker, M.K., White, N.A., Lessard, P., Thatcher, C.D., Pelzer, K.D., Davis, B. and Carmel, D.K., 1997. Prospective study of equine colic risk factors. Equine Vet Journal 29: 454-458.

Topliff, D.R., Potter, G.D., Dutson, T.R., Kreider, J.L. and Jessup, G.T., 1983. Diet manipulation and muscle glycogen in the equine. Proceedings equine Nutrition and Physiology Symposium 8, Lexington, KY, USA, pp. 224-229.

Topliff, D.R., Potter, G.D., Kreider, J.L., Dutson, T.R. and Jessup, G.T., 1985. Diet manipulation, muscle glycogen metabolism and anaerobic work performance in the equine. Proceedings equine Nutrition and Physiology Symposium 8, Lexington, KY, USA, pp. 119-124.

Van Weeren, P.R., 2006. Osteochondrosis In: Auer, J.A. and Stick, J.A. (eds,), Equine Surgery 3rd, Saunders Elsevier, St Louis, MO, USA, pp. 1166-1178.

Vander Heyden, L., Lejeune, J.P., Caudron, I., Detilleux, J., Sandersen, C., Chavatte, P., Paris, J., Deliège, B. and Serteyn, D., 2013. Association of breeding conditions with prevalence of osteochondrosis in foals. Veterinary Record 172: 68.

Vervuert, I. and Ellis, A., 2013. Developmental Orthopedic disease. In: Geor, R.J., Harris, P.A., Coenen, M. (eds.), Equine clinical and applied nutrition. Elsevier Inc, Philadelphia, PA, USA, pp. 536-548.

Waller, A.P. and Lindinger, M.I. 2010. Nutritional aspects of post exercise skeletal muscle glycogen synthesis in horses: A comparative review. Equine Veterinary Journal 42: 274-281.

Waller, A.P., Heigenhauser, G.J.F., Geor, R.J., L. and M.I., 2009. Fluid and electrolyte supplementation after prolonged moderate-intensity exercise enhances muscle glycogen resynthesis in horses. Journal of Applied Physiology 106: 91-100.

Wilke, A., Coenen, M., Distl, O., Hertsch, B., Christmann, L. and Bruns, E., 2003. Effect of locomotion on the development of osteochondrosis (OC) in Hannovarian Warmblood foals. In: Book of abstracts of the 54th Annual meeting of the European Association for animal Production. Wageningen Academic Publishers, Wageningen, the Netherlands, p. 392.

Willing, B., Vörös, S., Roos, S., Jones, A., Jansson, A. and Lindberg, J. E. 2009. Changes in faecal bacteria associated with concentrate and forage-only diets fed to horses in training. Equine Veterinary Journal 41: 908-914.

Zeyner, A. and Harris, P.A., 2013. Vitamins. In: Geor, R.J., Harris, P.A., Coenen, M. (eds.), Equine Clinical and Applied nutrition. Elsevier Inc, Philadelphia, PA, USA, pp. 168-189.

Oxidative stress in sport horses: Does it matter and if so, how should we feed them?

Carey A. Williams
Rutgers, the State University of New Jersey, Equine Science Center, Department of Animal Science, 84 Lipman Drive, New Brunswick, NJ 08901, USA; cwilliams@aesop.rutgers.edu

Take home message

Overall exercise studies have shown that oxidative stress was observed during endurance, intense, and treadmill exercise. The extent of the oxidative stress and muscle enzyme leakage was dependent on the ambient temperature, conditioning level and age of the horse, and the intensity of work. Supplementing antioxidants like vitamin E, vitamin C, and lipoic acid is beneficial to horses by decreasing the oxidative stress and muscle enzyme leakage, and increasing antioxidant status. Thus, we can provide better health and welfare to our equine athletes by supplementing with antioxidants before they are asked to perform under intense conditions. However, caution needs to be taken if supplementing above and beyond the recommended levels due to the possible interference with the absorption of other nutrients.

Introduction

Ever tried looking up '*oxidative stress*' on the Internet? Google brings up 8.6 million results; when adding '*horse*' to this search you get about 553,000. Try '*antioxidant*' and you get over 21 million results on Google (searches were done August 19, 2013). Either way you look at it, these are hot topics. A lengthy review has been published detailing oxidative stress and antioxidant supplementation in horses specifically and points out the many conflicting results (Kirschvink *et al.*, 2008). In the following article I will try to highlight studies from my laboratory along with other pertinent studies of oxidative stress in exercising horses and whether trials using antioxidant supplementation have been beneficial.

Oxidative stress background

The welfare of competing sport horses has attracted public attention following deaths at the Olympics and other championships. Welfare may be assessed partially by objective indicators of stress (heart rate, and various blood metabolites). Evidence of oxidative stress in horses has been described in reports dealing with intense (Chiaradia *et al.*, 1998; White *et al.*, 2001) and endurance exercise (Marlin *et al.*, 2002; Williams *et al.*, 2004a).

Oxidation provides energy for maintenance of cellular integrity and functions. Most of the consumed oxygen forms carbon dioxide and water, however, 1 to 2% of the oxygen is not completely reduced and forms reactive oxygen species (ROS). When antioxidant systems are insufficient, or when accumulation of ROS becomes chronic, oxidative processes may damage DNA, lipids, and contribute to degenerative changes, including aging and cancer. Lipids are protected directly by α-tocopherol (TOC) in the membranes and by other antioxidants, including ascorbic acid (ASC) in the cytosol or external spaces around cells.

It is important to note that ROS in moderation does play an important role in normal physiological activities. Production of superoxide by phagocytosing cells to kill invaded bacteria, up-regulation of endogenous defence systems to eliminate pro-carcinogens, and hydrogen peroxide can be considered a regulator of cell death pathways are a few examples (Franco *et al.*, 1999). In addition, during exercise ROS production may be required for normal force production in skeletal muscle, the development of training-induced adaptation in endurance performance, and the induction of endogenous defence systems (Powers *et al.*, 2010).

Antioxidants are inter-related and may prevent oxidant damage in several ways: scavenging of ROS; decreasing the conversion of less reactive ROS to more reactive ROS; facilitating repair of damage caused by ROS; and providing an environment favourable for activity of other antioxidants (Clarkson and Thompson, 2000). Lipid peroxidation occurs in tissues with a high concentration of poly-unsaturated fatty acids, such as cell and organelle membranes, lipoproteins, adipose tissue, and brain.

Antioxidant supplementation trials

Vitamin E and C

Vitamin E is the most commonly supplemented antioxidant in horses. One study found that a single bout of submaximal exercise does not affect plasma TOC concentration, but horses conditioned for several weeks, may require higher levels of vitamin E supplementation than recommended (Siciliano *et al.*, 1996).

It has been found in various species that vitamin C potentiates the effects of vitamin E by reducing the tocopheroxyl radicals and restoring its activity (Chan, 1993). Under maintenance conditions horses have the ability to synthesize sufficient ascorbate, but the demand increases as stress on the body is increased. One study looking at the vitamin E and C interaction used 40 endurance horses competing in an 80-km race for the purpose of research (Williams *et al.*, 2004b). Three weeks prior to the race the horses were provided with vitamin E (5,000 IU/d alpha-tocopheryl acetate) or vitamin E plus vitamin C (same vitamin E dose, plus 7 g ascorbic acid/d). The 27% increase in red blood cell (RBC) glutathione peroxidase (GPx) observed in the last two stages of this race in both treatment groups likely reflects a response to utilize reduced glutathione during the radical scavenging process (reduced glutathione donates an electron to reduce a wide variety of hydroperoxides using GPx as a catalyst). It also reflects the consumption of pro-oxidants generated during exercise. In contrast to the RBC changes, novel findings were the changes in the white blood cell (WBC) glutathione system. Fluctuations of WBC GPx during exercise and the sharp 41% increase during recovery may reflect replenishment of reduced glutathione. Compared to RBC, the higher concentration of WBC GPx and lower WBC total glutathione (GSH-T) may affect phagocyte oxidative burst and other immune functions during prolonged exercise.

Plasma ASC concentrations were lower in the horses supplemented with vitamin E alone than those receiving the vitamin E plus C at rest (Figure 1). This difference progressively diminished during the race as ASC increased in the vitamin E supplemented horses but remained unchanged in those also supplemented with C. This could be due to an increased mobilization of intracellular ASC stores when

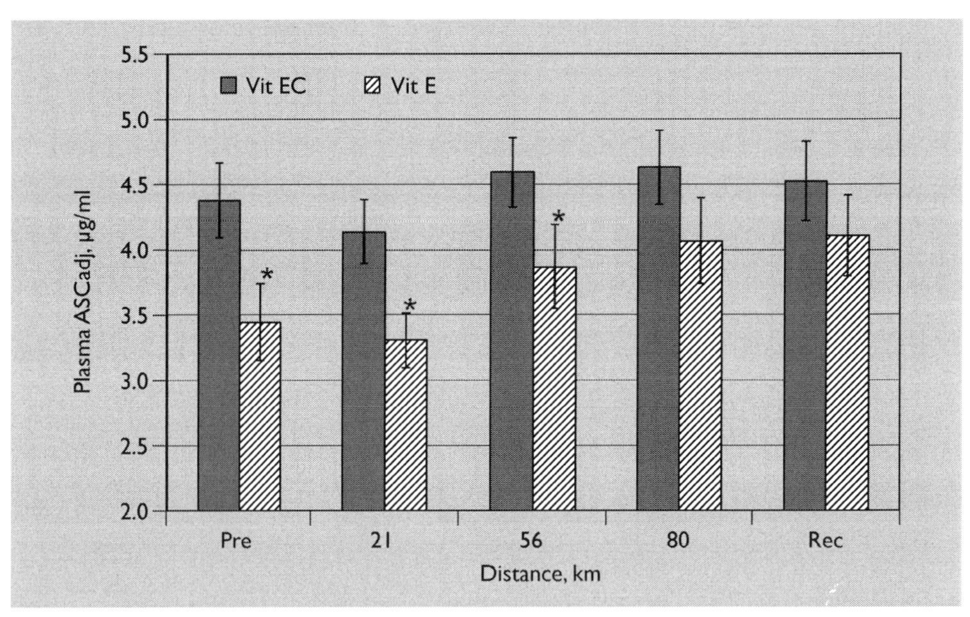

*Figure 1. Plasma ascorbate adjusted for albumin (ASCadj) for 34 horses completing an 80-km endurance ride in the vitamin E supplemented group (Vit E) and the vitamin E and C supplemented group (Vit EC) before (PRE), 21, 56, and 80 km during, and after recovery (REC) of an 80-km endurance race. *Treatments are significantly different at P<0.05 (Reprinted from Williams* et al., *2004b).*

supplemented with only vitamin E, whereas when adding C they were able to maintain ASC levels using the exogenous source for its antioxidant capacity. These findings contrast with a previous study, where a decrease in plasma ASC during a highly competitive and difficult 80 km race was found (Hargreaves *et al.*, 2003).

A study of polo ponies used similar vitamin E and C supplemented groups (Hoffman *et al.*, 2001). Throughout the polo season plasma TOC and ASC were higher in those also given vitamin C in hard-working ponies, but not those in only light work. These observations may reconcile the endurance findings where changes were observed in the highly competitive, mid-season race (Hargreaves *et al.*, 2003), but not in this lightly competitive, early season race (Williams *et al.*, 2004b). In a survey taken after the race, riders ranked the exertion level of the endurance ride easier than most of the rides later in the competition season. Also, ambient temperature was cooler in this race than in the summer when the majority of endurance competitions are held.

Vitamin E alone

Vitamin E intake was calculated in competitive endurance horses via a pre-ride survey detailing intake two weeks prior to the 80-km endurance race (Williams *et al.*, 2005). Pasture intake was estimated using 2.5% body weight eaten per day and subtracting amount of grain, hay, bran and/or other supplements obtained from the surveys. Horses were estimated to consume 1,150 to 4,700 IU/d of vitamin E in their total diet during this time period. This level is 1.2 to 5-times higher than the recommended levels given by the NRC (2007); which, at this intake, averages 1000 IU/d. The horses with the lower vitamin E intake generally were the horses receiving mostly pasture and minimal grain to supplement their diet. A negative correlation was found between the vitamin E intake and creatine kinase (CK), and aspartate aminotransferase (AST), and a positive correlation was found with intake and plasma TOC adjusted for albumin at all sample times. Enzyme activity in plasma is used as an indicator of muscle leakage during exercise. As apparent in the correlations found in the present study dietary intake of vitamin E is also a contributing factor in muscle enzyme plasma concentrations during exercise.

A negative correlation was found between finishing time and vitamin E intake for the 24 horses that finished the race (Williams *et al.*, 2005). One hypothesis for this finding could be that the higher placed horses were working at a greater intensity and/or being trained harder, thus having more sweet feed or supplements in the diet. Their higher level of conditioning may also have allowed these horses to work harder with lower muscle enzyme activities.

However, caution needs to be taken when supplementing with high levels of vitamin E. Other studies in my laboratory have investigated pharmaceutical levels of vitamin E on its impact of oxidative stress, muscle enzymes and antioxidant status (Williams and Carlucci, 2006). Horses supplemented with vitamin E at nearly 10-times the NRC (2007) recommended level did not experience lower oxidative stress compared to control horses (Williams and Carlucci, 2006). Additionally, there was found to be lower plasma β-carotene (BC) levels observed in this group compared to control or a moderately supplemented group, which may indicate that vitamin E, has an inhibitory effect on BC metabolism (Figure 2). This study failed to show that supplementation above control levels is more beneficial to oxidative stress and antioxidant status in intensely exercising horses. However, this research has proven that supplementing with levels in 10-times excess may be detrimental to BC and should be avoided.

Vitamin E and lipoic acid

Arabians trained to run on an equine treadmill were supplemented with vitamin E, lipoic acid (LA), or nothing (CON) before they underwent a simulated endurance exercise test of 3 exercise bouts totalling 55 km, with 20 min vet checks in-between (Williams *et al.*, 2004a). The results showed that apoptosis occurs in WBC during exercise and it can be moderated by supplementation with vitamin E or LA (Figure 3). The vitamin E group had 50% lower and the LA group had 40% lower

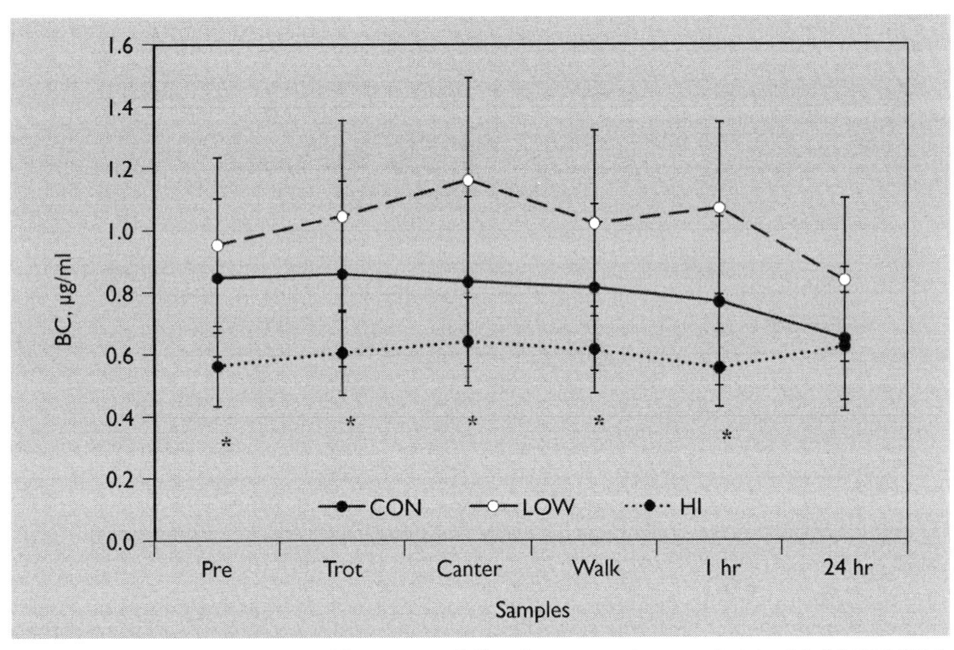

*Figure 2. Plasma concentrations of β-carotene (BC) in horses supplemented with a HI (10,000 IU/d), LOW (5,000 IU/d), or CON (no supplemental vitamin E) dose of vitamin E. * Indicates significant ($P<0.05$) difference between HI and LOW (Reprinted from Williams and Carlucci, 2006).*

apoptosis compared to the CON group. The increase in antioxidant status in the vitamin E and LA groups aided the WBC in scavenging the ROS triggering the apoptosis in these cells.

Antioxidants are linked together in various ways; this explains the increase in antioxidant status with supplementation of vitamin E and LA. In the present study LA increased the GSH-T concentrations in whole blood compared to CON (Williams *et al.*, 2004a). The LA group also had increased levels of ASC and TOC in the plasma throughout the study. Both the E and LA groups had about 40% more GSH-T, 30% more TOC, and 15% more ASC than the CON group. This illustrates recycling and scavenging of antioxidant radicals using the exogenous sources of the vitamin E and LA.

Superoxide dismutase

The effects of superoxide dismutase (SOD) on oxidative stress and inflammation in exercising horses systemically and locally (synovial fluid) was recently completed (Lamprecht *et al.*, 2012). Previous

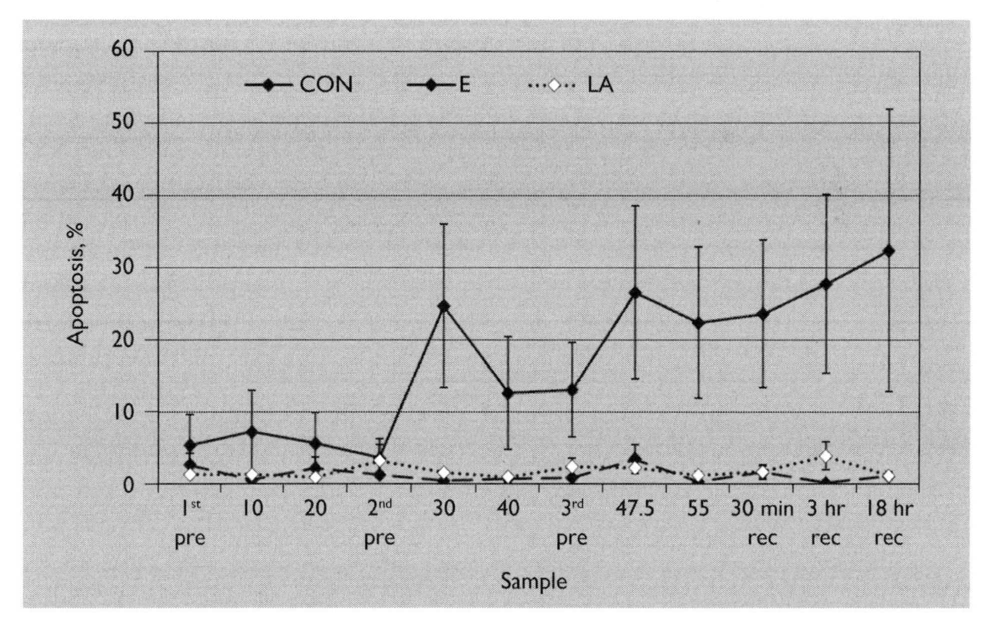

Figure 3. White blood cell apoptosis for the control (CON; n=3), vitamin E (E; n=3), and lipoic acid (LA; n=3) groups (Reprinted from Williams et al., *2004a).*

studies in rats (Radak *et al.*, 1995) and humans (Arent *et al.*, 2009, 2010) have shown beneficial results, however, these horse studies failed to show similar results. Horses supplemented with 3,000 IU of SOD for 6 weeks did not have a decrease in oxidative stress or an increase in antioxidant status including SOD activity as compared to those unsupplemented horses (Lamprecht *et al.*, 2012). However, studies have tested a SOD derivative on exhaustively exercising rats and found that it provided effective protection against oxidative stress in the liver and kidney along with skeletal muscle in exercising rats (Radak *et al.*, 1995). Recently, in humans, the effects of an oral SOD supplement on preseason collegiate soccer players (Arent *et al.*, 2010) and football players (Arent *et al.*, 2009) determined that performance improved by a greater magnitude in the soccer players supplemented with SOD, where the football players had greater improvements in peak power and lowered muscle breakdown, measured with CK, along with lower levels of 8-isoprostane.

Other exercise trials

Oxidative stress in old horses

Older horses are another group that might require antioxidant supplementation, especially if in combination with exercise. Developments in human molecular biology have supported the role of ROS production as a contributor to aging. The 'free radical theory of aging' states that long term effects of the degenerative changes associated with aging may create an accumulation of ROS and subsequent cellular damage and apoptosis (Harmon, 1956). In my laboratory we have found that evidence of a disequilibrium oxidant balance during exercise and aging showed varying results (Williams *et al.*, 2008). In old horses (22 ± 2 years), the amount of lipid peroxidation and blood antioxidant concentrations are similar to those found in mature but younger (12 ± 2 years) horses. Neither group had lipid peroxidation changes with either acute exercise or 8-weeks of training, but there was a higher concentration of total glutathione in the pre- vs. post-training tests in both age groups (Figure 4). The observation that more total glutathione was needed during the pre-training graded exercise test for both old and younger groups of horses suggests that training helped the horses prime their systems for the intense post-training exercise tests. Our study also found that WBC apoptosis was

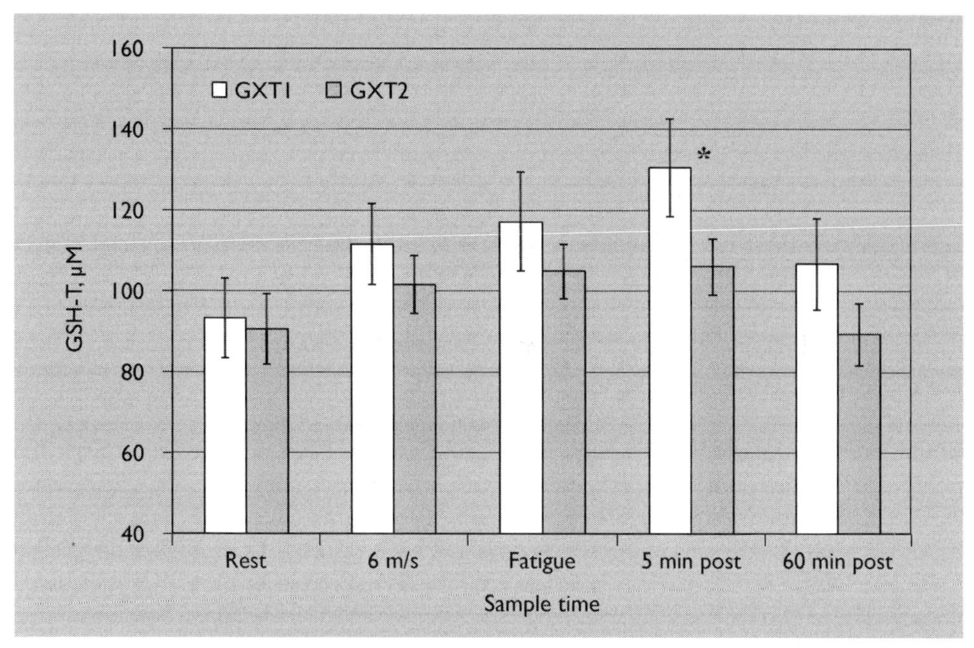

*Figure 4. Total red blood cell glutathione (GSH-T) concentrations for pre- and post-training (GXT1 and GXT2, respectively). The data from the mature and older horses have been combined due to lack of age group differences. * Indicates a difference between pre- and post-training tests (P<0.05; Reprinted from Williams* et al., *2008).*

significantly lower in the younger than in the older horses, signifying that age might have more of an impact on the immune system than on the oxidant/antioxidant system.

Oxidative stress in growing horses

Same as older horses that may require dietary intervention to help combat oxidative stress so might young growing horses that have just started their exercise training. However, many studies use already trained horses or horses in their 3 and 4-year old years. Recently studies have been performed using a group of Standardbred yearling fillies who have had nothing more than voluntary pasture exercise since birth (Smarsh, 2013). It was interesting that these studies showed that yearlings did not begin their exercise training with higher levels of oxidative stress in muscle or blood than mature mares as the authors originally hypothesized. The mares had higher lipid peroxidation and lower antioxidant status in the middle gluteal muscle prior to exercise training, implying that the mares had higher levels of oxidative stress overall. However, the older horses did improve their antioxidant status and oxidative stress levels at the completion of 8 weeks of exercise training, resulting in levels similar to the yearlings (Smarsh, 2013). This suggests that age alone was the biggest defence against increased oxidative stress after acute exercise and after exercise training in young growing horses.

Oxidative stress and three-day event competition

Elite three-day event horses competing internationally at a CCI** or CCI*** were the subjects for three different studies comparing nutritional status, inflammation, oxidative stress and antioxidant status before and after different phases of the competition. Detailed pre-event nutritional surveys were undertaken to determine the intake level of antioxidants and other nutrients that would affect the level of stress during competition (Burk and Williams, 2008; Williams and Burk, 2010). Results from the nutritional surveys can be found at Burk and Williams (2008). Through these surveys estimated daily intakes of vitamin E, K, Ca, P and Mg were calculated and found to be 2-4 times higher than daily recommended levels by the NRC (2007) (Williams and Burk, 2010). Also in response to competition, tumour necrosis factor-α, nitric oxide, and BC decreased, the muscle enzymes CK and AST increased, and TOC and retinol did not change throughout the study. The authors theorize that the training and conditioning programs of the horses and the elevated antioxidant and mineral intakes may have enhanced the horse's ability to modulate the inflammatory response and potential oxidative stress normally associated with rigorous bouts of acute exercise.

In another study, these high level competing horses were found to have no differences between the CCI** or CCI*** divisions for cortisol, TOC, retinol, BC, AST, and GPx (Williams and Burk, 2012). Total glutathione; however, was higher in the horses competing in the CCI** than horses in the CCI***. Total glutathione also peaked immediately after the cross-country phase returning to baseline after 18 to 24 hr of recovery. Other measures including CK, AST, GPx, BC, retinol, cortisol and lactate also peaked immediately after the cross-country phase and were typically lower before the competition started compared to 24 h after the cross-country. Overall these results provided the first report of antioxidant status of horses competing in either a CCI** and CCI*** 3-day event (Williams and Burk, 2010; 2012).

Even though there have been many studies examining the levels of lipid peroxidation, antioxidant status and other related metabolites or markers in the horse during exercise, we still have a long way to go before we fully understand the large variation in results both with and without antioxidant supplementation.

References

Arent, S.M., Davitt, P., Golem, D.L., Williams, C.A., McKeever, K.H. and Jaouhari, C., 2009. The effects of a post-workout nutraceutical drink on body composition, performance, and hormonal and biochemical responses in Division 1 college football players. Comp Exercise Physiol 6: 73-80.

Arent, S.M., Pellegrino, P.K., Williams, C.A., DiFabio, D. and Greenwood, J.C., 2010. Nutritional supplementation, performance, and oxidative stress in college soccer players. J Strength Cond Res 24: 1117-1124.

Burk, A.O. and Williams, C.A., 2008. Feeding management practices and supplement use in top level event horses. Comp Exercise Physiol 5: 85-93.

Chan, A.C., 1993. Partners in defense, vitamin E and vitamin C. Can J Physiol Pharmacol 71:725-731.

Chiaradia, E., Avellini, L., Rueca, F., Spaterna, A., Porciello, F., Antonioni, M.T. and Gaiti, A., 1998. Physical exercise, oxidative stress and muscle damage in race horses. Comp Biochem Physiol B 119: 833-836.

Clarkson, P.M. and Thompson, H.S., 2000. Antioxidants: what role do they play in physical activity and health? Am J Clin Nutr Suppl 72: 637S-646S.

Franco, A.A., Odom, R.S. and Rando, T.A., 1999. Regulation of antioxidant enzyme gene expression in response to oxidative stress and during differentiation of mouse skeletal muscle. Free Radic Biol Med 27: 1122-1132.

Hargreaves, B.J., Kronfeld, D.S., Waldron, J.N., Lopes, M.A., Gay, L.S., Saker, K.E., Cooper, W.L., Sklan, D.J. and Harris, P.A., 2003. Antioxidant status and muscle cell leakage during endurance exercise. Equine Vet J 34: 116-121.

Harmon, D., 1956. Aging: a theory based on free radical and radiation chemistry. J Gerontol 2: 298-314.

Hoffman, R.M., Morgan, K.L., Phillips, A., Dinger, J.E., Zinn, S.A. and Faustman, C., 2001. Dietary vitamin E and ascorbic acid influence nutritional status of exercising polo ponies. Equine Nutr Physiol Symp 17: 129-130.

Kirschvink, N., De Moffarts, B. and Lekeux, P., 2008. The oxidant/antioxidant equilibrium in horses. Vet J 177: 178-191.

Lamprecht, E.D. and Williams, C.A., 2012. Biomarkers of antioxidant status, inflammation, and cartilage metabolism are affected by acute intense exercise but not superoxide dismutase supplementation in horses. Oxid Med Cell Longev. doi: http://dx.doi.org/10.1155/2012/920932.

Marlin, D.J., Fenn, K., Smith, N., Deaton, C.D., Roberts, C.A., Harris, P.A., Dunster, C. and Kelly, F.J., 2002. Changes in circulatory antioxidant status in horses during prolonged exercise. J Nutr 132: 1622S-1627S.

NRC, 2007. Nutrient Requirements of Horses (6th ed.). National Academy Press, Washington, DC, USA.

Powers, S.K., Duarte, J., Kavazis, A.N. and Talbert, E.E., 2010. Reactive oxygen species are signaling molecules for skeletal muscle adaptation. Exp Physiol 95: 1-9.

Radak, Z., Asano, K., Inoue, M., Kizaki, T., Oh-Ishi, S., Suzuki, K., Taniguchi, N. and Ohno, H., 1995. Superoxide dismutase derivative reduces oxidative damage in skeletal muscle of rats during exhaustive exercise. J Appl Physiol 79: 129-135.

Siciliano, P.D., Parker, A.L. and Lawrence, L.M., 1996. Effect of dietary vitamin E supplementation on the integrity of skeletal muscle in exercised horses. J Anim Sci 75:1553-1560.

Smarsh, D.N., 2013. The impact of age and exercise on antioxidants and oxidative stress in horses. Doctoral Thesis. Rutgers, the State University of New Jersey. New Brunswick, NJ, USA.

White, A., Estrada, M., Walker, K., Wisnia, P., Filgueira, G., Valdes, F., Araneda, O., Behn, C. and Martinez, R., 2001. Role of exercise and ascorbate on plasma antioxidant capacity in Thoroughbred racehorses. Comp Biochem Physiol A 128: 99-104.

Williams, C.A. and Burk, A.O., 2010. Nutrient intake during an elite level three-day eventing competition is correlated to inflammatory markers and antioxidant status. Equine Vet J Suppl 42: 116-122.

Williams, C.A. and Burk, A.O., 2012. Antioxidant status in elite three-day event horses during competition. Oxid Med Cell Longev. DOI: http://dx.doi.org/10.1155/2012/572090.

Williams, C.A. and Carlucci, S., 2006. Oral vitamin E supplementation and oxidative stress, vitamin and antioxidant status in intensely exercising horses. Equine Vet J Suppl 36: 617-621.

Williams, C.A., Gordon, M.B., Betros, C. and McKeever, K.H., 2008. Apoptosis and antioxidant status are influenced by age and exercise training in horses. J Anim Sci 86: 576-583.

Williams, C.A., Kronfeld, D.S., Hess, T.M., Saker, K.E. and Harris, P.A., 2004a. Lipoic acid and vitamin E supplementation to horses diminishes endurance exercise induced oxidative stress, muscle enzyme leakage, and apoptosis. In: Lindner, A. (ed.) The elite race and endurance horse. CESMAS, Oslo, Norway, pp. 105-119.

Williams, C.A., Kronfeld, D.S., Hess, T.M., Saker, K.E., Waldron, J.N. and Harris, P.A., 2005. Vitamin E intake and systemic antioxidant status in competitive endurance horses. Equine Comp Exercise Physiol 2: 149-152.

Williams, C.A., Kronfeld, D.S., Hess, T.M., Waldron, J.N., Crandell, K.M., Saker, K.E., Hoffman, R.M. and Harris, P.A., 2004b. Antioxidant supplementation and subsequent oxidative stress of horses during an 80-km endurance race. J Anim Sci 82: 588-594.

Lessons from the feeding of human athletes: nutritional modulation of muscle during training and rehabilitation

Ron J. Maughan
School of Sport, Exercise and Health Sciences, Loughborough University, Loughborough, LE11 3TU, United Kingdom; r.j.maughan@lboro.ac.uk

Take home message

Diet can significantly influence athletic performance, for better or for worse. The food choices that an athlete makes can support consistent, intensive and effective training while minimising the risk of chronic fatigue, illness and injury. Specific strategies before and during competition will depend on the nature of the sport and on the physiological and metabolic characteristics of the individual. Athletes also need to pay particular attention to their energy and nutrient needs during periods of injury and rehabilitation: the reduced energy intake necessary to prevent unwanted weight gain must be balanced against the need to prevent large losses of lean tissue mass. Supplements are generally not necessary, but targeted use of a few supplements may have benefits. Hydration is an important consideration: small losses of body water are well tolerated, but losses of more than about 2% of body mass may impair performance.

Introduction

Those who succeed at the highest level of sports competition owe the major part of their success to three key factors. The first is their genetic endowment, which provides them with the physical, physiological and metabolic characteristics that predispose to success in their chosen event: the strength and power athlete has very different physiological and metabolic characteristics from the endurance athlete. The second factor, which amplifies these differences, is a sustained period of intensive training. The third factor is psychological: an intense desire to win, coupled with a willingness to tolerate, and even embrace, the rigours of the training program. In elite sport, however, all of the competitors are more or less equally matched with regard to these characteristics, and so they look to other factors that can provide a performance advantage. It is not surprising therefore that sportsmen and women generally are concerned about their diet, although this concern is not always matched by an understanding of current knowledge in the area of nutrition. Some of the dietary practices followed by athletes in pursuit of success are sound, but others have no beneficial effect and may even be harmful. As in other areas of nutrition, these ideas are often encouraged by those who stand to gain financially from sales of dietary supplements. Athletes also tend to follow the practices of successful competitors, even when these are clearly not the reasons for their success.

Two distinct aspects of the athlete's nutrition program must be considered; the first is the diet in training which must be consumed on a daily basis for a large part of the year, and the second is the diet in the immediate pre-competition period and during competition itself. Considering the range of activities encompassed by the term sport and the variation in the characteristics of the individuals taking part, it is not surprising that the nutritional requirements vary. For recreational activities, and for the individual who exercises for health reasons, the daily diet forms part of a lifestyle that may be quite different from that of the competitive athlete, but the nutritional implications of exercise participation apply equally, albeit to different degrees.

There is now a growing realisation that eating strategies for athletes must take account of the fact that each individual has different nutrition goals. At the elite level in sport, it is not acceptable any more to make generic prescriptions for all members of a team or for all competitors in any event. A strategy must be devised to take account of each athlete's physiological and biochemical characteristics as well as the training load and competition goals.

Nutrition for training

A key issue for the athlete during training is to meet the additional nutrient requirement imposed by the training load. In sports involving prolonged strenuous exercise on a regular basis, participation has a significant effect on energy balance. Metabolic rate during training for running or cycling, for example, may be 15-20 times the resting rate, and such levels of activity may be sustained for several hours each day. Evidence suggests that the metabolic rate may remain elevated for at least 12 and possibly up to 24 hours if the exercise is prolonged and close to the maximum intensity that can be sustained; this has been disputed, and it is unlikely that metabolic rate remains elevated for long periods after more moderate exercise. If body weight and performance levels are to be maintained, the high rate of energy expenditure must be matched by a high energy intake. Available data for most athletes suggest that they are in energy balance within the limits of the techniques used for measuring intake and expenditure, though there are some who seem to be in chronic low energy availability (Loucks, 2013). This is to be expected as a chronic deficit in energy intake would lead to a progressive loss of body mass. However, data for women engaged in sports where a low body weight, and especially a low body fat content, are important, including events such as gymnastics, distance running and ballet, consistently show a lower than expected energy intake (Loucks, 2007). There is no obvious physiological explanation for this finding other than methodological errors in the calculation of energy intake and expenditure, but it seems odd that these should apply specifically to this group of athletes. Many of these women do, however, have a very low body fat content: a body fat content of less than 10% is not uncommon in female long distance runners. Secondary amenorrhoea, possibly related more to the training regimen than to the low body fat content, is common in these women, but is usually reversed when training stops (Manore *et al.*, 2007).

Not every athlete needs a high energy intake, however. Technical sports such as gymnastics may involve many hours of technique training but with a low overall energy demand. A low energy intake need not imply an inadequate energy intake, but it does limit the intake of all nutrients, and athletes with low energy intakes must be more careful to select foods that will meet all their nutrient requirements. We are also learning to balance the performance benefits of a low body mass and low body fat content with the potential for long term harm to health (Lohman *et al.*, 2012).

Protein

Athletes engaged in strength and power events have traditionally been concerned with achieving a high dietary protein intake in the belief that this is necessary for muscle growth and repair. In a survey of American college athletes, 98% believed that a high protein diet would improve performance. While a diet deficient in protein will lead to loss of muscle tissue, there is no evidence to support the idea that excess dietary protein will drive the system in favour of protein synthesis, though there remains a lively debate about how much protein is necessary for muscle growth in athletes (Phillips and van Loon, 2011). Excess protein will simply be used as a substrate for oxidative metabolism, either directly or as a precursor of glucose, and the excess nitrogen will be lost in the urine. Exercise, whether it is long distance running, aerobics or weight training, will cause an increased protein oxidation compared with the resting state (Millward, 2003). The fractional contribution of protein oxidation to energy production during the exercise period may decrease to about 5% of the total energy requirement, compared with about 10-15% (i.e. the normal fraction of protein in the diet) at rest, but the absolute rate of protein degradation is increased during exercise because of the high metabolic rate. This leads to an increase in the minimum daily protein requirement, but, at least for most individuals, this will be met if a normal mixed diet adequate to meet the increased energy expenditure is consumed. In spite of this, however, many athletes ingest large quantities of protein containing foods and expensive protein supplements; daily protein intakes of up to 400 grams are not unknown in some sports. There also remains the issue of those who restrict energy intake to maintain a low body mass and the restricted energy intake that applies during periods of injury. Even if an increase in the absolute amount of protein consumed is not necessary, a change in the food choices to ensure a greater fractional contribution of protein to total energy intake is likely to be necessary.

The timing of protein intake relative to training may be more important than the amount of protein consumed (Phillips and Van Loon, 2011). Remodelling of the muscle tissues takes place in the hours and days after the training stimulus has been applied: consumption of small amounts of protein can ensure positive protein balance. As little as 6 gram of essential amino acids, or about 20 gram of high quality mixed protein, ingested either just before or soon after training may help promote adaptations taking place within the muscles (Glover and Phillips, 2010). Resistance training in the fasted state and without ingesting some protein-containing foods soon after training will not optimise the training response. Milk protein, which is high in leucine, may be more effective than some other proteins in promoting net muscle glycogen synthesis after a resistance training session (Phillips *et al.*, 2009).

Carbohydrate

The energy requirements of training are largely met by oxidation of fat and carbohydrate. The higher the intensity of exercise, the greater the reliance on carbohydrate as a fuel: at an exercise intensity corresponding to about 50% of an individual's maximum oxygen uptake (VO_{2max}), approximately two thirds of the total energy requirement is met by fat oxidation, with carbohydrate oxidation supplying about one third (Romijn *et al.*, 1993). If the exercise intensity is increased to about 75% of VO_{2max}, the total energy expenditure is increased, and carbohydrate is now the major fuel. If carbohydrate is not available, or is available in only a limited amount, the intensity of the exercise must be reduced to a level where the energy requirement can be met by fat oxidation.

The primary need for endurance athletes, therefore, is for the carbohydrate intake to be sufficient to enable the exercise load to be sustained at the high level necessary to produce a response. During each strenuous exercise session, substantial depletion of the glycogen stores in the exercising muscles and in the liver takes place. Sprinters and team sports athletes, whose training often involves repeated short sprints, may also experience substantial depletion of the muscle glycogen stores. In a sprint lasting 10-60 s, the major part of the energy demand is met by the conversion of muscle glycogen to lactate. Though some of the lactate can be salvaged by the liver for gluconeogenesis, a substantial part is oxidised and is thus not available for glycogen resynthesis. If the muscle carbohydrate reserve is not replenished before the next training session, training intensity must be reduced, leading to corresponding decrements in the training response. Any athlete training hard on a daily basis can readily observe this; if a low carbohydrate diet, consisting mostly of fat and protein, is consumed after a day's training, it will be difficult to repeat the same training load on the following day.

Feeding a high fat, low carbohydrate diet for periods lasting from a few days to a few weeks has been shown to increase the capacity of muscle to oxidise fat (Hawley and Burke, 2010). This can certainly improve endurance capacity in the rat, but may not be as effective in man. Similarly, short term fasting increases endurance capacity in the rat, but results in a decreased exercise tolerance in man (Burke, 2010). The training diet, therefore should be high in carbohydrate, with a large proportion of total energy intake in the form of complex carbohydrates and simple sugars. Rather than thinking of carbohydrate needs as a fraction of total energy intake, it may be better to prescribe intakes in absolute terms relative to body mass (Burke *et al.*, 2011). Thus, an intake of 6-10 g/kg body mass may be necessary for athletes training hard. Some long exercise sessions should perhaps be performed in a fasted or carbohydrate-depleted state to maximise the capacity for fat oxidation, but athletes should probably ensure that carbohydrate stores are replete for high intensity exercise sessions. These high levels of intake are difficult to achieve without consuming large amounts of simple sugars and other compact forms of carbohydrate: as well as increasing the frequency of meals and snacks towards a 'grazing' eating pattern. Athletes may find that sugar, jam, honey and high sugar foods such as confectionery, as well as carbohydrate-containing drinks, such as soft drinks, fruit juices and specialist sports drinks, can provide a low-bulk, convenient addition of carbohydrate to the nutritious food base. There is no evidence that this pattern of eating is harmful for those with high levels of energy expenditure; for the individual who has to fit an exercise programme into a busy day, it is inevitable that changes to eating patterns must be made, but these need not compromise the quality of the diet.

Failure to meet carbohydrate needs may also make the athlete more susceptible to a variety of minor infectious illnesses. Exercising with low carbohydrate reserves can result in increased levels of stress hormones, particularly cortisol, which in turn impairs the functional capacity of the immune system. While usually trivial in themselves, these illnesses can disrupt training and may prevent participation in important competitions (Robson-Ansley *et al.*, 2009).

Micronutrients and dietary supplements

With regular strenuous training, there must be an increased total intake to balance the increased energy expenditure. Provided that a reasonably varied diet is consumed, this will generally supply more than adequate amounts of protein, minerals, vitamins and other dietary requirements. There is no good evidence to suggest that specific supplementation with any of these dietary components is necessary or that it will improve performance. Athletes who chronically restrict energy intake to limit body mass, and especially fat mass, may benefit from a broad spectrum vitamin and mineral supplement. Athletes with limited finances, little interest in the foods they eat, or lacking in food preparation skills may also fail to consume a varied diet. While supplements are no substitute for good dietary choices, they may have a use in some of these situations.

The only exceptions to the generalisation about the value of dietary supplements for meeting micronutrient needs may be iron, vitamin D, and, in the case of very active women, calcium. Highly trained endurance athletes commonly have low circulating haemoglobin levels, although total red cell mass may be elevated due to an increased blood volume. This may be considered to be an adaptation to the trained state, but hard training may result in an increased iron requirement and exercise tolerance is impaired in the presence of anaemia. Low serum folate and serum ferritin levels are not associated with impaired performance, however, and correction of these deficiencies does not influence indices of fitness in trained athletes (Ljungqvist *et al.*, 2009). Moderate weight-bearing exercise has been reported to increase bone mineral density in women, and this may be a significant benefit of exercise for most women: hard training, however, may reduce circulating oestrogen levels and hence accelerate bone loss. For these athletes, an adequate calcium intake should be ensured, although calcium supplements themselves will not reverse bone loss while oestrogen levels remain low. It must be emphasised that iron or calcium supplements should only be taken on the advice of a qualified practitioner after suitable investigative procedures have indicated an inadequate intake. Even then, alternatives to supplementation, specifically alterations in the selection of foods to achieve a higher intake must also be considered. Low fat dairy produce, for example, is a good source of calcium in an energy restricted diet. The issue of whether athletes should supplement with vitamin D is at present controversial, though the argument seems to be moving in favour of supplementation. While arguments for and against vitamin D supplementation exist, there is growing evidence that many athletes are vitamin D deficient or insufficient, especially those who train indoors, who wear protective clothing while outdoors or who live at high latitudes (Larson-Meyer and Willis, 2010). Although there is not good evidence that routine vitamin D supplementation is beneficial to athletes, there is some evidence from cross-sectional studies of an association between circulating vitamin D levels and athletic performance (Cannell *et al.*, 2009). It therefore seems prudent to recommend that athletes seek professional help to monitor their serum vitamin D concentration.

A concern with many supplements on sale – apart from the lack of evidence of efficacy and safety – is the recent spate of reports of contamination of supplements with prohibited substances, including stimulants and anabolic steroids (Maughan, 2005). The amounts present are generally too small to be effective in improving performance, but can cause a positive drugs test (Watson *et al.*, 2009). In some cases, however, high doses – even higher than the normal therapeutic dose – of steroids, stimulants and anorectic agents have been found in supplements, with not only potential performance benefits but with a real risk of adverse health effects. One of the best-selling supplements – hydroxycut – was withdrawn from sale in 2009 because of links with liver damage that reportedly led to at least one fatality (Seminerio and Sweetser, 2010).

Hydration

Many athletes never drink during exercise, often because of the difficulties of access to drinks. Drinking, however, may be useful in reducing the sensation of effort and in improving the quality of training sessions. The skill of drinking also needs to be practised and where athletes will drink during competition it is useful to become familiar with the sensation of exercising with fluid in the gut. There may be other advantages from ensuring good hydration during and after each exercise session (Maughan and Meyer, 2013). Cell volume is an important regulator of metabolic processes, and there may be opportunities to manipulate this to promote anabolic processes in muscle and other tissues. During and after exercise there may be large changes in cell volume, secondary to osmotic pressure changes caused by metabolic activity, hydrostatic pressure changes, or by sweat loss (Watson and Maughan, 2013). Alterations in cell volume induced by changes in osmolality are well known to alter the rate of glycogen synthesis in skeletal muscle (Lang *et al.*, 1998). Amino acid transport into muscles is also affected by changes in cell volume induced by manipulation of the trans-membrane osmotic gradient: skeletal muscle uptake of glutamine is stimulated by cell swelling and inhibited by cell shrinkage (Lang 2011). The intracellular glutamine concentration appears to play an important role in a number of processes, including protein and glycogen synthesis, but the effect of ingestion of glutamine on these aspects of post-exercise recovery is not known at this time. The full significance of these findings for the post-exercise recovery process and the roles they play in adaptation to a training program remain to be established. Manipulation of fluid and electrolyte balance and the ingestion of a variety of osmotically active substances or their precursors offers potential for optimising the effectiveness of a training regimen, but the current state of knowledge does not allow definitive guidance on this.

Nutrition for competition

The ability to perform prolonged exercise can be substantially modified by dietary intake in the pre-exercise period, and this becomes important for the individual aiming to produce peak performance on a specific day. Dietary manipulation to increase muscle glycogen content in the few days prior to exercise has been extensively recommended for endurance athletes following observations that these procedures were effective in increasing endurance capacity in cycle ergometer exercise lasting about 1.5-2 h. The suggested procedure was to deplete muscle glycogen by prolonged exercise about one week prior to competition and to prevent resynthesis by consuming a low carbohydrate diet for 2-3 days before changing to a high carbohydrate diet for the last 3 days during which little or no exercise was performed. This procedure can double the muscle glycogen content and is effective in increasing cycling or running performance. There is now a considerable amount of evidence that it is not necessary to include the low carbohydrate glycogen depletion phase of the diet for endurance athletes. It is commonly recommended that it is sufficient to reduce the training load over the last few days before competition and to simultaneously increase the dietary carbohydrate intake (Burke *et al.*, 2011). This avoids many of the problems associated with the more extreme forms of the diet. However, there is some evidence that the inclusion of a bout of hard exercise followed by a low-carbohydrate phase prior to a few days of a high-carbohydrate diet may confer metabolic, and perhaps also performance, benefits (Shinihara *et al.*, 2010). Although an increased pre-competition muscle glycogen content is undoubtedly beneficial, there is a faster rate of muscle glycogen utilisation when the glycogen content itself is increased, thus nullifying some of the advantage gained.

A high carbohydrate diet in the days prior to competition may also benefit competitors in games such as rugby, soccer or hockey, although it appears not to be usual for these players to pay attention to this aspect of their diet. In one study, players starting a soccer game with low muscle glycogen content did less running, and much less running at high speed, than those players who began the game with a normal muscle glycogen content (Saltin, 1973). It is common for players to have one game in midweek as well as one at the weekend, and it is likely that full restoration of the muscle glycogen content will not occur between games unless a conscious effort is made to achieve a high carbohydrate intake.

The muscle (and liver) glycogen loading procedure is generally restricted to use by athletes engaged in endurance events, but the muscle glycogen content may influence performance in events lasting only a few minutes (Maughan and Poole, 1981). It is clear that low muscle glycogen stores will impair the capacity for high intensity exercise. A high muscle glycogen content may be particularly important when repeated sprints at near maximum speed have to be made.

A wide range of supplements is on sale to athletes, often with exaggerated claims of efficacy in enhancing performance in competition. Many of these are not supported by evidence of either their effects on performance or their safety when taken in high doses for prolonged periods (Maughan *et al.*, 2007). Sports supplements which may be useful in helping the athlete meet nutritional goals during training and competition include sports drinks, high carbohydrate supplements and liquid meal supplements. These are more expensive than everyday foods, but often provide a convenient and practical way of meeting dietary needs in a specific situation. There is good evidence for an ergogenic effect of a few supplements in some specific situations, including caffeine, creatine, and bicarbonate or other buffering agents, possibly including β-alanine. Caffeine in relatively small doses – typically 2-4 mg/kg – can improve performance in a variety of exercise tasks, with greater effects generally seen in prolonged exercise, probably by actions on adenosine receptors in the central nervous system rather than on lipolysis as was previously thought (Davis *et al.*, 2003). Creatine – in the form of creatine phosphate – acts as an energy source for ATP resynthesis in high intensity exercise. Meat eaters normally obtain about 1 gram per day from their diet, which is about 50% of the daily requirement, with the remainder synthesised from amino acids. Ingestion of about 10-20 g of creatine for a period of 4-6 days can increase the muscle creatine content by 10-20%, leading to improvements in strength and sprint performance (Kreider, 2003). The biggest improvements in performance are generally seen in repeated sprints with limited recovery. Acute ingestion of large doses of sodium bicarbonate (about 0.3 g/kg) can increase the extracellular buffering capacity and improve performance in exercise lasting from about 30 s to about 10 minutes. Similar benefits may be seen from a few days of β-alanine supplementation, which leads to an increase in muscle carnosine content and hence in buffer capacity (Sale *et al.*, 2010). Recent data suggest a beneficial effect on exercise performance of large doses of dietary nitrate, which have been shown to reduce the oxygen cost of exercise (Larsen *et al.*, 2007; 2011) and to improve performance (Bailey *et al.*, 2009). Both inorganic nitrate and vegetable sources, such as beetroot juice, have been shown to be effective.

There is scope for nutritional intervention during exercise only when the duration of events is sufficient to allow absorption of drinks or foods ingested and where the rules of the sport permit. The primary aims must be to ingest a source of energy, usually in the form of carbohydrate, and fluid for replacement of water lost as sweat. High rates of sweat secretion are necessary during hard exercise in order to limit the rise in body temperature which would otherwise occur. If the exercise is prolonged, this leads to progressive dehydration and loss of electrolytes. Fatigue towards the end of a prolonged event may result as much from the effects of dehydration as from substrate depletion.

Beginning exercise in a dehydrated state is certainly harmful to performance of high intensity exercise (Goulet *et al.*, 2010) and to endurance performance (Gigou *et al.*, 2010).

The composition of drinks to be taken before and during exercise should be chosen to suit individual circumstances (Maughan and Shirreffs, 2008). Sweat rates and sweat composition vary greatly between individuals, so prescription of fixed rates of fluid intake is generally not helpful. During exercise in the cold, fluid replacement may not be necessary as sweat rates will be low (though sweat rates may still be substantial if heavy clothing is worn), but there remains a need to supply additional glucose to the exercising muscles. Consumption of a high-carbohydrate diet in the days prior to exercise should reduce the need for carbohydrate ingestion during exercise in events lasting less than about 2 hours, but it is not always possible to achieve this; competition on successive days, for example, may prevent adequate replacement of liver and muscle glycogen stores between exercise periods. In this situation, more concentrated glucose drinks are to be preferred, and recent evidence supports the inclusion of glucose/fructose mixtures when high rates of carbohydrate delivery are needed (Jeukendrup, 2010). These will supply more glucose thus sparing the limited glycogen stores in the muscles and liver without overloading the body with fluid. In many sports there is little provision for fluid replacement: participants in games such as football or hockey can lose large amounts of fluid, but replacement is possible only at the half time interval. Cold drinks can enhance endurance performance in warm weather more effectively than warm drinks by acting as a heat sink to slow the rate of rise of core temperature (Lee *et al.*, 2008a,b). Most athletes finish endurance events with some degree of dehydration, but some slower performers may consume fluid in excess of sweat losses. This is not helpful to performance and may in extreme cases lead to hyponatraemia, which is occasionally fatal (Hew-Butler *et al.*, 2008).

Sports drinks containing glycerol – which acts to expand the plasma volume – have been popular with some endurance athletes, but as of January 1, 2010, these fall within the prohibited list of the World Anti-Doping Agency, so their use in competition is not permitted (WADA, 2010). Many other compounds have similar effects as a result of their osmotic properties, though, and it remains to be seen whether these will also be prohibited on the basis that they act through similar mechanisms.

In the post-exercise period, replacement of fluid and electrolytes can usually be achieved through the normal dietary intake. If there is a need to ensure adequate replacement before exercise is repeated, extra fluids should be taken and additional salt (sodium chloride) might usefully be added to food. It is noteworthy that the composition of sweat varies greatly between individuals, with the sodium content of sweat ranging between about 10 and 80 mmol/l (Schirreffs and Maughan, 1997). The other major electrolytes, particularly potassium, magnesium and calcium, are present in abundance in fruit and fruit juices. Salt or mineral supplements are not normally necessary, though some cases of muscle cramp may be associated with high salt losses and may be prevented by ingestion of drinks with moderate-high salt content (Stofan *et al.*, 2005).

Conclusion

Recent developments in sports nutrition research have substantially changed the nutrition practices of athletes, but communication of new research findings to athletes can take time. It is also clear that there is a large variability in the individual physiological and metabolic characteristics of athletes that make it difficult to give generic advice. Metabolic profiling of athletes, which has been proposed over the last 20 years, is likely to be overtaken by genetic profiling which offers opportunities for identifying the gene-nutrient interactions that dictate the adaptations that take place in response to training. This will allow better integration of training and nutrition on an individualised basis. New dietary supplements continue to appear and it is impossible to predict what new developments will take place in this area, but better screening of these compounds for both efficacy and safety will be necessary.

References

Bailey, S.J., Winyard, P., Vanhatalo, A., Blackwell, J.R., DiMenna, F.J., Wilkerson, D.P., Tarr, J., Benjamin, N. and Jones A.M., 2009. Dietary nitrate supplementation reduces the O_2 cost of low-intensity exercise and enhances tolerance to high-intensity exercise in humans. Journal of Applied Physiology 107: 1144-1155

Burke, L.M., 2010. Fueling strategies to optimize performance: training high or training low? Scandinavian Journal of Medicine and Science in Sports Suppl. 20: 11-21.

Burke, L.M., Hawley, J.A., Wong, S. and Jeukendrup, A.E., 2011. Carbohydrates for training and competition. Journal of Sports Sciences 29: S17-S27.

Cannell, J,J,, Hillis, B.W., Sorenson, M.B., Taft, T.N. and Anderson, J.J.B., 2009. Athletic performance and vitamin D. Medicine and Science in Sports and Exercise 41: 1102-1110.

Davis, J.M., Zhao, Z.W. and Stock, H.S., 2003. Central nervous system effects of caffeine and adenosine on fatigue. American Journal of Physiology 284: R399-R404

Gigou, P.-Y., Lamontagne-Lacasse, M. and Goulet, E.D.B., 2010. Meta-analysis of the effects of pre-exercise hypohydration on endurance performance, lactate threshold and VO_2max. Medicine and Science in Sports and Exercise 42: S254.

Glover, E.I. and Phillips, S.M., 2010. Resistance exercise and appropriate nutrition to counteract muscle wasting and promote muscle hypertrophy. Current Opinion in Clinical Nutrition and Metabolic Care 13: 630-634.

Goulet, E.D.B., Lamontagne-Lacasse, M., Gigou, P.-Y., Kenefick, R.W., Ely, B.R. and Cheuvront, S., 2010. Pre-exercise hypohydration effects on jumping ability and muscle strength, endurance and anaerobic capacity: a meta-analysis. Medicine and Science in Sports and Exercise 42: S254.

Hawley, J.A. and Burke, L.M., 2010. Carbohydrate availability and training adaptation: Effects on cell metabolism and exercise capacity. Exercise and Sport Science Reviews 38: 152-160.

Hew-Butler, T., Ayus, J.C., Kipps, C., Maughan, R.J., Mettler, S., Meeuwisse, W.H., Page, A.J., Reid, S.A., Rehrer, N.J., Roberts, W.O., Rogers, I.R. Rosner, M.H., Siegel, A.J., Speedy, D.B., Stuempfle, K.J., Verbalis, J.G., Weschler, L.B. and Wharam, P., 2008. Consensus Statement of the 2nd International Exercise-Associated Hyponatremia Consensus Development Conference. Clinical Journal of Sports Medicine 18: 111-121.

Jeukendrup, A.E. 2010. Carbohydrate and exercise performance: the role of multiple transportable carbohydrates. Current Opinion in Clinical Nutrition and Metabolic Care 13: 452-457.

Kreider, R.B., 2003. Effects of creatine supplementation on performance and training adaptations. Molecular and Cellular Biochemistry 244: 89-94.

Lang, F., 2011. Effect of cell hydration on metabolism. In: Maughan, R.J., Burke, L.M. (eds.) Sports nutrition: more than just calories – triggers for adaptation. Nestlé Nutr Inst Workshop Ser; Karger AG, Basel, Switzerland, 69: 131-149.

Lang, F., Busch, G.L., Ritter, M., Völkl, H., Waldegger, S. and Gulbins, E., 1998. Functional significance of cell volume regulatory mechanisms. Physiological Reviews 78: 247-306.

Larsen, F.J., Schiffer, T.A., Bourniquet, S., Sahlin, K. Ekblom, B., Lundberg, J.O. and Weitzberg, E., 2011. Dietary inorganic nitrate improves mitochondrial efficiency in humans. Cell Metabolism 13, 149-159.

Larsen, F.K., Ekblom, B., Sahlin, K., Lundberg, J.O. and Weitzberg, E., 2007. Effects of dietary nitrate on oxygen cost during exercise. Acta Physiologica 191: 59-66.

Larson-Meyer, D.E. and Willis, K.S., 2010. Vitamin D and athletes. Current Sports Medicine Reports 9: 220-226.

Lee, J.K.W., Maughan, R.J. and Shirreffs, S.M., 2008a. The influence of serial feeding of drinks at different temperatures on thermoregulatory responses during cycling. Journal of Sports Sciences 26: 583-590.

Lee, J.K.W., Shirreffs, S.M. and Maughan, R.J., 2008b. Cold drink ingestion improves exercise endurance capacity in the heat. Medicine and Science in Sports and Exercise 40: 1637-1644.

Ljungqvist, A., Jenoure, P., Engebretsen, L., *et al.*, 2009. The International Olympic Committee (IOC) Consensus Statement on periodic health evaluation of elite athletes March 2009. International Sportmedicine Journal 10: 124-144.

Lohman, T., Ackland, T., Sundgot-Borgen, J., Maughan, R.J., Meyer, N., Stewart, A. and Mueller, W., 2012. Current status of body composition assessment in sport. Sports Medicine 42: 227-249.

Loucks, A.B., 2007. Low energy availability in the marathon and other endurance sports. Sports Medicine 37: 348-352:

Loucks, A.B., 2013. Energy balance and energy availability. In: Maughan, R.J. (ed.) Nutrition in sports. Wiley-Blackwell, Oxford, in press.

Manore, M.M., Kam, L.C. and Loucks, A.B., 2007. The female athlete triad: Components, nutrition issues, and health consequences. Journal of Sports Sciences 25: S61-S71.

Maughan R.J. and Meyer, N.L., 2013. Hydration during intense exercise training. In: Van Loon, L.J.C., Meeusen, R. (eds.) Limits of Human Endurance. Nestlé Nutr Inst Workshop Ser, 76: 25-37.

Maughan, R.J. and Poole, D.C., 1981. The effects of a glycogen loading regimen on the capacity to perform anaerobic exercise. European Journal of Applied Physiology 46: 211-221.

Maughan, R.J. and Shirreffs, S.M., 2008. Development of individual hydration strategies for athletes. International Journal of Sport Nutrition and Exercise Metabolism 18: 457-472.

Maughan, R.J., 2005. Contamination of dietary supplements and positive drugs tests in sport. Journal of Sports Sciences 23: 883-889.

Maughan, R.J., Depiesse, F. and Geyer, H., 2007. The use of dietary supplements by athletes. Journal of Sports Sciences 25: S103-S113.

Millward, D.J., 2003. An adaptive metabolic demand model for protein and amino acid requirements. British Journal of Nutrition 90: 249-260.

Phillips, S.M. and Van Loon, L.J.C., 2011. Dietary protein for athletes: from requirements to optimum adaptation. Journal of Sports Sciences 29: S29-S38.

Phillips, S.M., Tang, J.E. and Moore, D.R., 2009. The role of milk- and soy-based protein in support of muscle protein synthesis and muscle protein accretion in young and elderly persons. Journal of the American College of Nutrition 28: 343-354.

Robson-Ansley, P.J., Gleeson, M. and Ansley, L., 2009. Fatigue management in the preparation of Olympic athletes. Journal of Sports Sciences 27: 1409-1420.

Romijn, J.A., Coyle, E.F., Sidossis, L.E., Gastaldelli, A., Horowitz, J.F., Endert, E. and Wolfe, R.R., 1993. Regulation of endogenous fat and carbohydrate metabolism in relation to exercise intensity and duration. American Journal of Physiology 265: E380-E391.

Sale, C., Saunders, B. and Harris, R.C., 2010. Effect of beta-alanine supplementation on muscle carnosine concentrations and exercise performance. Amino Acids 39: 321-333.

Saltin, B., 1973. Metabolic fundamentals in exercise. Medicine and Science in Sports 5: 137-146.

Seminerio, J. and Sweetser, S., 2010. Drug Induced Liver Injury Secondary to Hydroxycut. American Journal of Gastroenterology 105: S270.

Shinihara, A., Takakura, J., Yamane, A. and Suzuki, M. 2010. Effect of the Classic 1-Week Glycogen-Loading Regimen on Fat-Loading in Rats and Humans. Journal of Nutrition Science and Vitaminology 56: 299-304.

Shirreffs, S.M. and Maughan, R.J., 1997. Whole body sweat collection in man: an improved method with some preliminary data on electrolyte composition. Journal of Applied Physiology 82: 336-341.

Stofan, J.R., Zachwieja, J.J. and Horswill, C.A., 2005. Sweat and sodium losses in NCAA football players: A precursor to heat cramps? International Journal of Sport Nutrition and Exercise Metabolism 15: 641-652.

WADA, 2010. The World Anti-Doping Agency prohibited list, 2010. Accessed at: http://www.wada-ama.org/Documents/World_Anti-Doping_Program/WADP-Prohibited-list/WADA_Prohibited_List_2010_EN.pdf

Watson, P. and Maughan, J.J., 2013. Artifacts in plasma volume changes due to hematology analyzer derived hematocrit. Medicine and Science in Sports and Exercise, in press.

Watson, P., Houghton, E., Grace, P.B., Judkins, C., Dunster, P.M. and Maughan, R.J., 2009. Excretion pattern of nandrolone metabolites after ingestion of a nandrolone pro-hormone: effects of delivery mode. Medicine and Science in Sports and Exercise 41: 766-772.

Protein ingestion and utilisation in performance horses related to muscle adaptation for conditioning and regeneration

Manfred Coenen
Institute of Animal Nutrition, Nutrition Diseases and Dietetics, An den Tierkliniken 9, 04103 Leipzi, Germany; coenen@vetmed.uni-leipzig.de

Introduction

On the first view, muscle activity is linked to energy supply to the cell. This is quite logical as the shortening of the myosin units is strictly dependent on the presence of adenosintriphophate (ATP). Many experimental as well as practical studies are focussed on energy metabolism in exercising horses since the second half of the 19th century up to nowadays (Bauedement 1852; Goachet *et al.*, 2010; Jansson and Lindberg, 2012; Lovell, 1985; Müntz, 1880; Von Engelhardt, 1992). The results of the highly recognized study of Fick and Wislicenus (Fick und Wislicenus, 1868; Kleiber, 1961) who climbed the Swiss mountain 'Faulhorn' in order to measure energy turnover and in particular the protein catabolism, are intensively used to conclude that protein turnover is not involved in the metabolism of exercising muscle tissue. An additional general suggestion is that dietary protein is not limiting muscle performance. Regardless of those statements, meanwhile it is accepted to recommend a protein intake of about 1.25-2-fold of maintenance level for human athletes (Lemon *et al.*, 1984; Tarnopolsky, 2004).

The protein requirement in exercising horses is not well defined. The aim of this article is to force a discussion on protein requirements for performance horses.

Protein evaluation

Although 'protein' is the common term to communicate intake and fate of nitrogenous compounds it is misleading or even false. The animal's organism requires amino acids (AA) which are delivered by dietary AA and/or internal synthesis. Of course, the crude proten (CP) in feedstuff is represented mostly by AA but CP gives no precise information about the AA provision due to several reasons:

1. The AA-profile (AA in g/100 g protein) is different among feedstuffs.
2. The CP in some feeds contains free AA or other non-protein-nitrogen (NPN); most important are feedstuffs with added urea - illegal manipulation of total nitrogen (N).
3. The AA-profile of feedstuffs is not identical to the required AA-profile; the endogenous AA synthesis balances the dietary AA as far as the essential AA are not limiting.
4. Neither the CP nor the apparently digestible CP define the AA uptake of monogastric animals including equids. Gastric pepsin – activated by the acidic gastric environment – and the proteolytic capacities deriving from pancreatic secretion and mucosa of the small intestine (SI) ensure the presentation of peptides and AA to the mucosal surface in SI. These compounds are absorbed in the SI by roughly 90% independent of the quantity in CP intake (Zeyner *et al.*, 2010; Gfe, 2013). The AA which reach the hindgut are indigestible or decomposed by microbial activity. The product of microbial driven hindgut protein degradation is ammonia. Ammonia permeates easily through the gut wall. The viscera drainage ensures the ammonia disposal towards the liver and urea synthesis transforms the toxic ammonia to non-critical urea. There is no valid contribution of hindgut nitrogen absorption to the AA-pool of the metabolism (Urschel und Lawrence, 2013).

The nitrogen in feedstuff can be divided in two major compartments: (1) cell-wall fraction and (2) cell content. A survey of literature data shows that the N in the neutral detergent fibre fraction (NDF) is a sufficient estimate of cell wall associated N (Zeyner *et al.*, 2010) representing that part of N that is not assessable for digestion in SI. Consequently, the difference between total N and NDF-N refers to the precaecally digestible protein ($CP_{SI\text{-}dig}$), mostly from the plant cell content. The absorption of this protein fraction is rather uniform by 90% (Zeyner *et al.*, 2010). Hereby, the precaecal digestible AA are defined as the AA-profile in this fraction, and this fraction is almost identical with the AA-profile of the total CP that is described by common tables on feed composition.

This model enables to evaluate the $CP_{SI\text{-}dig}$ and $AA_{SI\text{-}dig}$ in any feedstuff by the common analytical procedures. Although the described system gives the estimate about the AA in a specific feedstuff that are presented to the precaecal absorption it should be noted that the process of intraluminal protein degradation and mucosal uptake is not based on individual single AA. The majority of AA are absorbed via tri- or dipeptides (Urschel und Lawrence, 2013). This phenomenon only is adequate for protein/AA evaluation and calculation of AA-requirement. Differences in precaecal absorption between the $AA_{SI\text{-}dig}$ will be limited.

Protein/Amino acid requirement

The protein/AA-requirement is defined by quantity of product protein, AA in the protein of the product and the utilisation of (precaecally) absorbed AA. This is quite simple in case of lactation but rather difficult in case of other conditions:

- Prenatal growth: the AA accretion in the conceptus is not the complete explanation for protein/AA requirements in mares. There exists an enormous exchange of AA via placental tissue and the feto-placental unit use of AA as a resource for energy.
- Muscle activity: the conversion of chemical energy from digested feed and body stores into kinetic energy is a simple description of exercise related increases in energy requirements of exercising horses. The morphologic structures that are involved in the kinetic energy used for performance are build by proteins; the metabolic tools ensuring the energy conversion are proteins. So far, there is essentially a big role for proteins in exercising muscle tissue and in principle an exercise related need for protein or AA respectively.

Considering the principles valid regardless of quantity aspects, the needs of protein or AA for exercise are linked to:

1. Adaptation of muscle tissue (response on training).
   - enlargement of muscle cells; this needs to be associated to an increase in stored proteins as the protein content of muscle tissue in trained horses is maintained or even elevated;

   - increased budget of enzymes like citrate synthase;
   - increase of mitochondrial mass.
2. Cellular function during exercise.
   - Cori cycle and alanine cycle: these metabolic processes enable to derive energy anaerobically from pyruvate leaving lactate, shuttling the lactate and ammonium to the liver and powering recycling of carbon skeletons for the muscle cell;
   - desamination of amino acids and oxidation of the carbon skeleton for production of ATP (*Peters et al.*, 2013);
   - protein leakage of muscle cells during exercise.
3. Tissue recovery and repair after exercise.
   - tissue damage is a physiological side effect of exercise;
   - the tissue restores the protein stores and up regulates protein synthesis (Aguirre *et al.*, 2013; Edgett *et al.*, 2013; Matsui *et al.*, 2006; Van den Hoven *et al.*, 2010).

These aspects indicate that protein/AA are essentially linked to muscle activity and that this tissue may respond to oral intake of proteins (Urschel und Lawrence, 2013). However the question on the quantity that is needed in exercising horses above maintenance level awaits an answer.

The plasma AA in exercising horses responds to dietary supplementation (Urschel *et al.*, 2010) and may maintain or even increase muscle mass (Urschel *et al.*, 2010). The data shows that a specific AA supplementation induces metabolic changes in exercising horses and therefore the hypothesis that additional AA provided post exercise may improve recovery of muscle tissue including the restoration of energy stores can be postulated. However, the hypothesis may be limited to horses with high physical exercise workload (endurance horses, 3-day-eventers). Literature data of other species shows that muscle mass can be maintained better with enforced AA supply within a defined time slot after exercise. This seems to be linked to a specific signalling cascade ('mammalian target of rapamycine', mTOR) that regulates muscle tissue protein synthesis (Urschel und Lawrence, 2013). Leucine is involved in this process. Interestingly milk protein, a limiting factor for postnatal muscle growth, has a relatively high concentration of this AA. Milk protein (casein), soy or linseed protein can serve as AA sources. But again, there is a lack on equine data regarding AA as a muscle performance-modifying factor.

Protein intake by common diets

Typical, appropriate diets contain more than 12% of CP in dietary dry matter (DM) and the DM-intake at 2-3% of body weight (BW) easily results in a protein ingestion at 2fold of maintenance requirement. Diets consisting of 80% average hay (12% CP/kg) and 20% of cereals will provide ~135 g CP/kg DM or ~93 g $CP_{SI\text{-}dig}$/kg DM. A DM-intake of 2.5% of BW will result in a $CP_{SI\text{-}dig}$ intake of around three times the maintenance level. Based on these data it is unlikely that the AA-supply by average diets can be a performance limiting factor. But again, there is a lack on equine data regarding AA as a muscle performance-modifying factor.

Empirically it seems that poor hay (>10% CP) may be poorly digested precaecally and therefore reduce AA digestion too. But such hay qualities are well accepted or even preferred in practice. Protein excess is blamed to depress performance. In fact, high protein ingestion increases the urea level in blood and increases the need for disposal of non-used nitrogen. Protein excess can elevate water intake due to the enforced diuresis and augmented renal losses of phosphorus. Those effects are debatable at >18% of CP in dietary DM.

The risks of low-protein-diets in exercising horses are underestimated in the feeding practice. Forages low in CP are low in precaecally digestible AA and are likely inadequate in young horses at the onset of training when the growth of the muscle tissue is more important and the adaptation of the tissue to training is required.

References

Aguirre, N., Van Loon, L.J. and Baar, K., 2013. The role of amino acids in skeletal muscle adaptation to exercise. Nestle Nutrition Institute Workshop Series 76: 85-102.

Bauedement, E., 1852. Études expérimentales sur l'alimentation du bétail. Annales de l'Institut agronomique 4: 158-163.

Edgett, B.A., Fortner, M.L., Bonen, A. and Gurd, B.J., 2013. Mammalian target of rapamycin pathway is up-regulated by both acute endurance exercise and chronic muscle contraction in rat skeletal muscle. Applied Physiology and Nutrition Metabolism 38: 862-869.

Fick, A. and Wislicenus. J., 1868. Recherches sur l´origine de la force musculaire. Annales des Sciences Narurelle; 5. série; Zoologie, Paleonthologie: 257-279.

Gesellschaft für Ernährungsphysiologie der Haustiere (GFE), 2013. Empfehlungen zur Energie- und Nährstoffversorgung des Pferdes. Frankfurt/Main, DLG-Verlag. In Press.

Goachet, A.G., Varloud, M., Philippeau, C. and Julliand, V., 2010. Long-term effects of endurance training on total tract apparent digestibility, total mean retention time and faecal microbial ecosystem in competing Arabian horses. Equine Veterinary Journal Supplement: 387-392.

Jansson, A. and Lindberg, J.E., 2012. A forage-only diet alters the metabolic response of horses in training. Animal 6: 1939-1946.

Kleiber, M., 1961. The fire of life. John Wiley & Sons, Hoboken, USA.

Lemon, P.W., Yarasheski, K.E. and Dolny, D.G.,1984. The importance of protein for athletes. Sports Medicine 1: 474-484.

Lovell, D.K., 1985. Exercise physiology. An overview. Veterinary Clinics of North America Equine Practice 1: 439-445.

Matsui, A., Ohmura, H., Asai, T., Takahashi, T., Hiraga, A., Okamura, K., Tokimura, H., Sugino, T., Obitsu, T. and Taniguchi, K., 2006. Effect of amino acid and glucose administration following exercise on the turnover of muscle protein in the hindlimb femoral region of thoroughbreds. Equine Veterinary Journal Supplement 38: 611-616.

Müntz, A., 1880. Recherches sur la digestion des fourrages employeés dans l'alimentation des chevaux. De la digestibilité des fourrages donnés isolement. Institute National Agronomique. Paris, France: 195-227.

Peters, L.W., Smiet, E., de Sain-van der Velden, M.G., and van der Kolk, J.H., 2013. Amino acid utilization by the hindlimb of warmblood horses at rest and following low intensity exercise. Veterinary Quarterly 33: 20-24.

Tarnopolsky, M., 2004. Protein requirements for endurance athletes. Nutrition 20: 662-668.

Urschel, K.L., Geor, R.J., Waterfall, H.L., Shoveller, A.K. and McCutcheon, L.J., 2010. Effects of leucine or whey protein addition to an oral glucose solution on serum insulin, plasma glucose and plasma amino acid responses in horses at rest and following exercise. Equine Veterinary Journal Supplement: 347-354.

Urschel, K.L. and Lawrence, L.M., 2013. Amino acids and protein. In: Equine applied and Clinical Nutrition. Geor, R.J., Harris, P.A. and Coenen, M. (Eds.). Elsevier Publishers. Edinburgh, United Kingdom.

Van den Hoven, R., Bauer, A., Hackl, S., Zickl, M., Spona, J. and Zentek, J. ZENTEK, 2010. Changes in intramuscular amino acid levels in submaximally exercised horses - a pilot study. Journal of Animal Physiology Animaml Nutrition 94: 455-464.

Von Engelhardt, W., 1992. Physical performance – a comparison between horses and men. Deutsche Tierärztliche Wochenschrift 99: 24-26.

Zeyner, A., Kirchhof S. Susenbeth, A., Sudekum, K.H. and Kienzle, E., 2010. Protein evaluation of horse feed: a novel concept. In: Ellis, A.D., Longland, A.C., Coenen, M. and Miraglia, N. (eds.) The impact of nutrition on the health and welfare of horses. EAAP Publication no. 128. Wageningen Academic Publishers, Wageningen, the Netherlands, pp. 40-42.

Influence of the rider skills, balance and athletic condition on the performance ability of horses

Lars Roepstorff
Department of Anatomy, Physiology and Biochemistry, Unit of Equine Studies, Swedish University of Agricultural Sciences, P.O. Box 7011, 750 07 Uppsala, Sweden; lars.roepstorff@slu.se

Introduction

For a vast majority of owners soundness and performance of the horse are two very important key terms. No matter if the horse is intended for sport, work or leisure we want them to perform well while staying sound. The most common cause of veterinary consultation and also culling of horses are orthopaedic injuries. A very important symptom of these injuries is locomotion asymmetry caused by pain. Asymmetry could also be caused by the rider. So what affects the performance and soundness of the horse?

This is an extremely complex interaction between many factors (Figure 1). To achieve good performance with sustainable soundness you firstly need to understand that loading is the cause of both training effect and injury. Without loading muscles, supportive tissues and the circulatory system the horse will not get stronger or a better performer. At the same time it is always overload in relation to the prerequisites of the horse and its present training status that causes a majority of orthopaedic injuries, i.e. training injuries. It is overloading, irrespectively if it is a temporary overload causing a fracture or a sprained ligament or if it is more long-term minor overload, that causes wear and tear injury such as osteoarthritis or tendinitis. Slight over-load could be due to everything from poor conformation and gait to training, poor riding, arena surfaces, farriery and so on. So, which *factors* determine loading?

The most basic functional factors are speed, strength, endurance and technique. Technique could be gait of the horse as well as specific

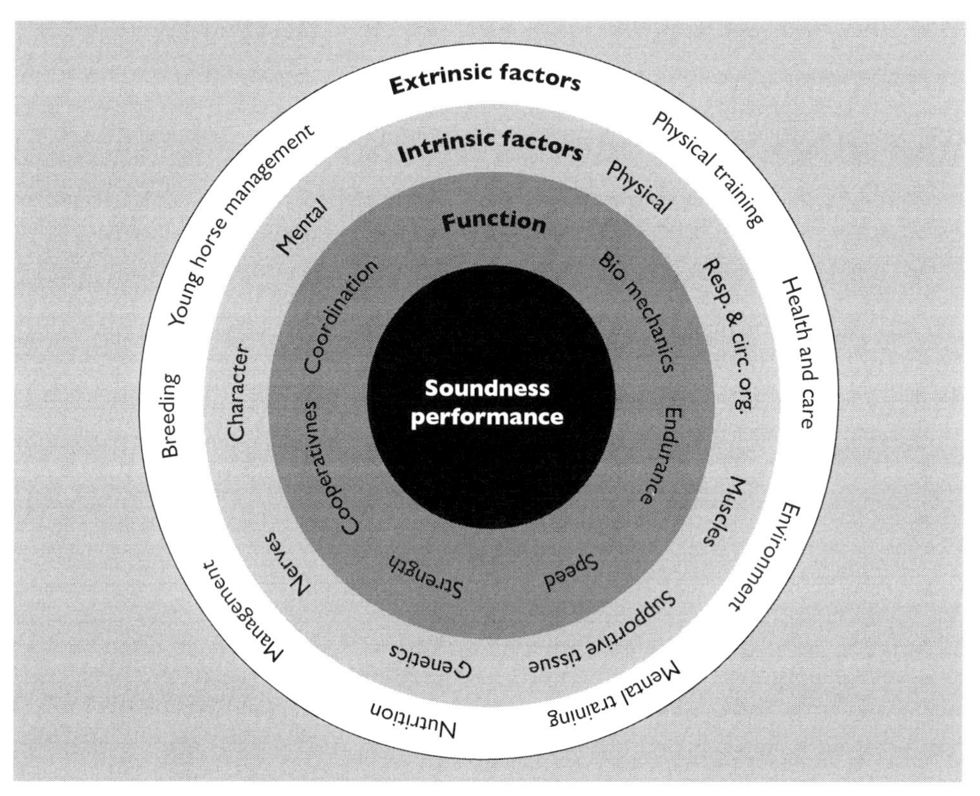

Figure 1. The many factors affecting the soundness and performance of (sports) horses.

movement patterns. It could also be called biomechanics or simply movement of the horse. Additionally the cooperativeness and the coordination are important functional factors affecting load on the whole locomotor apparatus. All these things vary a lot depending on what you want to do, racing, show jumping, western riding, endurance, dressage, riding school work, etc. This is a basic reason for preferring different conformation, gait and mental properties of the horse, but also to take care and train it in different ways and on different surfaces.

Next level of factors could be called intrinsic factors, which is anatomy and physiology. It is basically about understanding the most vital organs and tissues involved in performance but also how and why they are affected by orthopaedic injuries. Strictly speaking the whole body is involved in performance but here we present the ones most important for locomotion. The infrastructure of the horse is the skeleton, cartilage, ligaments and tendons also called supportive tissues. These are also the ones affected when we talk about orthopaedic injuries. Next, muscles are used to propel the infrastructure and the circulatory and respiratory organs (heart lungs, blood) provide oxygen to the muscles so they can transform oxygen and fuel (the metabolised food) into dynamic work. Again the characters as well as the nerves, the connection between brain, spinal cord and muscles are important. We might also mention the genes that determine all of the above.

The third level of factors could be characterized as extrinsic factors and are those that we can affect by our way of interacting with the horse. Probably the most important is how we train the horse: amount, intensity and type of training hugely affect loading of the locomotor apparatus and therefore both performance and risk of orthopaedic injury. Other things are health and care of the horse, i.e. how we prevent and take care of diseases and injuries, everything from vaccination and health checks to antiparasitic programs, shoeing, trimming and mouth inspections, the mental training or education of the horse, how and what we feed. How we house and keep our horses, the environment, which is everything from stable ventilation to the surfaces we are training on and breeding is the way we influence the genes. You might say that young horse management and training are also very important, but strictly it is all above during a specific part of the life.

Rider influence on horse locomotion

The large majority of the equine insurance claims, both for veterinary care and mortality are due to locomotor problems (Egenvall *et al.*, 2006; Penell *et al.*, 2005). Back problems constitute a common reason for euthanasia (Egenvall *et al.*, 2006). The composition and magnitude of the training have been found to be risk factors for unsoundness (Egenvall *et al.*, 2013), while others have specifically targeted the riding (Greve and Dyson, 2013a,b), identifying that crooked riders were associated with lame horses.

Lameness and asymmetry in horse

The exact problem in a horse with relatively mild clinical lameness often remains undetermined, accordingly most often also its cause.

Greve and Dyson (2013a), using subjective lameness investigation, found that in horses with lameness the saddle had often slipped to one side, which made the rider sit in a crooked position (Greve and Dyson, 2013a,b). They could also abolish the lameness and the saddle slip after analgesia in nearly all horses. However, horses as well as humans, are born with sidedness (Murphy *et al.*, 2005), which will to some degree complicate the decision of whether to label a horse as lame or only asymmetric.

Asymmetry in general and in humans

Sidedness has been studied quite extensively in humans, e.g. there is even a scientific journal named *Journal of Laterality*. Humans also show relatively grave asymmetries (20%) compared to horses (2%) (Weishaupt *et al.*, 2004). The goal is to ride your horse straight (Anonymous 2002: 139). One interpretation is that a horse working straight should work and show suppleness at equal amounts to the left and right side. As horses are being trained by basically much-more asymmetrical beings, the potentially large rider-induced symmetries deserve focus.

Riding and the seat

Riding is communication with the horse through various aids: the voice, the hand, the seat, the leg, the whip or the voice, even if the seat is by many thought of as the most important aid. One reason for its importance can be that it is always there, once mounted, i.e. taking away the rein actions or diminishing the influence of the legs is simpler/possible, but as long as the weight is placed on the horse it is there and must be managed. Equestrian literature has throughout history emphasized the importance of a correct seat and good balance for good performance in horseback riding (Anonymous, 2002).

A number of scientific studies have addressed the rider's seat. These studies mainly involved a general description of the seat (Byström *et al.*, 2009) and how riders changed their movement pattern when becoming more educated in riding (Kang *et al.*, 2010; Schils *et al.*, 1993; Terada *et al.*, 2006). The classical seat for a rider has been defined: the axis is the rider's ischium and the ear, shoulder, waist, and heel should form an imaginary straight line (Kang *et al.*, 2010; Lovett *et al.*, 2003).

The studies have identified both common (Byström *et al.*, 2009) and rider and horse specific movement patterns (Schöllhorn *et al.*, 2006). However, experienced riding instructors failed to reach consensus with respect to specific deviations from the correct seat (Blokhuis-Zetterquist *et al.*, 2008). This warrants more in depth biomechanical studies on individual postural strategies of riders. Postural control has been defined as the ability to control the body in space and ensure its stability and orientation (Brodal, 2004).

Back locomotion can be investigated by skin fixated markers (Faber *et al.*, 2001). With this technique it has been shown that the changes in rider seat can significantly change back locomotion pattern of the horse (Roepstorff *et al.*, 2009).

We have investigated sagittal seat data from seven riders on a treadmill (Byström *et al.*, 2009; Weishaupt *et al.*, 2006). Three postural strategies were distinguished, using individual-level kinematic data from pelvis, trunk and head. The strategies correlated to subjective evaluation of rider posture. The results indicated that rider asymmetries or postural deficits could be categorized quantitatively. Another observation from this project (Byström *et al.*, 2009; Weishaupt *et al.*, 2006) is that the horses became more and more asymmetric when the riders strived to affect them to an increased degree (unpublished observations).

There is scientific evidence that foot pronation (rotational movement of the foot at the subtalar and talocalcaneonavicular joints) influences dynamic postural control of humans, not only in the lower limb. It could affect all the way up to pelvis. In a study at Strömsholm riding school 28 students were selected based on having or not having foot pronation. When two experienced riding teachers evaluated the 28 students blindly there was a highly significant difference in assessed seat quality between the groups with versus without foot pronation (Elkaer *et al.*, 2013).

The rider as an athlete

It is likely that if the seat could be taught in a more evidence-based way, with the basics anchored more into rider-targeted science, there is potential for improvement in the riders posture, both on elite and non-elite level. Just presently some Olympic nations have also started using physiotherapists for their riders, in order to increase health and performance in both riders and horses, but in general there is a perception that relative to other sports the body of the rider is somewhat neglected both for performance and health. In addition, the prevalence of back pain in riders has been studied and found to be even higher (88%), than the estimate for the general population (60-80%; Kraft *et al.*, 2007; Lövquist *et al.*, 2009). To match the gaited horses of today riders as well as veterinarians working with orthopaedic health of the horse need strategies and increased knowledge about the rider influence on the horse.

Food for future thoughts

As has been discussed rider skills may have considerable impact on horse locomotion and thereby long term health. This raises two important questions. Could horses be misdiagnosed and treated for orthopaedic injuries that are basically a physiological adaptation to being trained by an asymmetric rider (causing an asymmetrical locomotion pattern in the horse)? Do horses get orthopaedic injuries due to being trained by an asymmetric rider? The prerequisite to answer these questions is more knowledge about rider asymmetry and its influence on horse locomotion!

References

Anonymous, 2002. Principles of riding. Official Instruction Handbook of the German National Equestrian Federation. Kenilworth Press, Wykey, UK.

Blokhuis-Zetterqvist, M., Aronsson, A., Hartmann, E., Van Reenan, C. and Keeling, L., 2008 Assessing riders seat and horses behaviour. Difficulties and perspectives. Journal of Applied Animal Welfare Science 11: 191-203.

Brodal, P., 2004. Det nevrobiologiske grunnlaget for balanse [Neurological basis of balance]. Fysioterapeuten 8: 25-30.

Byström, A., Rhodin, M., Peinen, K., Weishaupt, M.A. and Roepstorff, L., 2009. Basic kinematics of the saddle and rider in high-level dressage horses trotting on a treadmill. Equine Veterinary Journal 41: 280-284.

Egenvall, A., Penell, J.C., Bonnett, B.N., Olson, P. and Pringle J., 2006. Mortality of Swedish horses with complete life insurance between 1997 and 2000 – variations with sex, age, breed and diagnosis. Veterinary Record 158: 397-406.

Egenvall, A., Tranquille, C.A., Lönnell, A.C., Bitschnau, C., Oomen, A., Hernlund, E., Montavon, S., Franko Andersson, M., Murray, R.C., Weishaupt, M.A., van Weeren, R. and Roepstorff, L., 2013. Days-lost to training and competition in relation to workload in 263 elite show-jumping horses in four European countries. Preventive Veterinary Medicine, in press.

Elkjaer, L.P., Rohrwacher, L. and Roesberg, S., 2013. Överpronation kopplad till ryttarens sits. Available at: http://stud.epsilon.slu.se/5735/7/ploug_elkjaer_etal_130625.pdf.

Faber, M., Schamhardt, H., Van Weeren, R. and Barneveld, A., 2001. Methodology and validity of assessing kinematics of the thoracolumbar vertebral column in horses on the basis of skin-fixated markers. American Journal of Veterinary Research 62: 301-306.

Greve, L. and Dyson, S.J., 2013a. An investigation of the relationship between hindlimb lameness and saddle slip. Equine Veterinary Journal 45: 570-577.

Greve, L. and Dyson, S., 2013b. The horse-saddle-rider interaction. Veterinary Journal 195: 275-281.

Kang, O.D., Ryu, Y.C., Ryew, C.C., Oh, W.Y., Lee, C.E. and Kang, M.S., 2010. Comparative analyses of rider position according to skills levels during walk and trot in Jeju horse. Human Movement Science 29: 956-963.

Kraft, C.N., Urban, N., Ilg, A., Wallny, T., Scharfstädt, A., Jäger, M. And Pennekamp, P.H., 2007. Influence of the riding discipline and riding intensity on the incidence of back pain in competitive horseback riders. Sportverletzungen Sportschaden 21: 29-33.

Lagarde, J., Kelso, J.A., Peham, C. and Licka, T., 2005. Coordination dynamics of the horse-rider system. Journal Motility Behaviour 37: 418-424.

Lovett, T., Hodson-Tale, E. and Nankervis, K., 2005. A preliminary investigation of rider position during walk, trot and canter. Equine and Comparative Exercise Physiology 2: 71-76.

Löfqvist, L., Pinzke, S., Stål, M. and Lundqvist, P., 2009. Riding instructors, their musculoskeletal health and working conditions. Journal of Agricultural Safety and Health 15: 241-254.

Murphy, J., Sutherland, A. and Arkins, S., 2005. Idiosyncratic motor laterality in the horse. Applied Animal Behaviour 90: 297-305.

Penell, J.C., Egenvall, A., Bonnett, B.N., Olson, P. and Pringle, J., 2005. Specific causes of morbidity among Swedish horses insured for veterinary care between 1997 and 2000. Veterinary Record 157: 470-477.

Roepstorff, L., Egenvall, A., Rhodin, M., Byström, A., Johnston, C., Weeren, P. R. and Weishaupt, M., 2009. Kinetics and kinematics of the horse comparing left and right rising trot. Equine Veterinary Journal 41: 292-296.

Schils, S.J., Greer, N.L., Stoner, L.J. and Kobluk, C.N., 1993. Kinematic analysis of the equestrian walk, posting trot and sitting trot. Human Movement Science, 12: 693-712.

Schöllhorn, W.L., Peham, C., Licka, T. and Scheidl, M., 2006. A pattern recognition approach for the quantification of horse and rider interaction. Equine Veterinary Journal 36 Supplement: 400-405.

Symes, D. and Ellis, R., 2009. A preliminary study into rider asymmetry within equitation. Veterinary Journal 181: 34-37.

Terada, K., 2000. Comparison of head movements and EMG activity of muscles between advanced and novice horseback riders at different gaits. Journal of Equine Science 11: 83-90.

Weishaupt, M.A., Wiestner, T., von Peinen, K., Waldern, N., Roepstorff, L., van Weeren, R., Meyer, H. and Johnston, C., 2006. Effect of head and neck position on vertical ground reaction forces and interlimb coordination in the dressage horse ridden at walk and trot on a treadmill. Equine Veterinary Journal 36 Supplement: 387-392.

Weishaupt, M.A., Wiestner, T., Hogg, H.P., Jordan, P. and Auer, J.A., 2004. Vertical ground reaction force-time histories of sound Warmblood horses trotting on a treadmill. Veterinary Journal 168: 304-311.

How to train tendons in human athletes

Adamantios Arampatzis, Sebastian Bohm and Falk Mersmann
Humboldt-University Berlin, Department of Training and Movement Sciences, Philippstraße 13, Haus 11, 10115 Berlin, Germany; a.arampatzis@hu-berlin.de

Fundamentals of tendon mechanics

Mechanical properties of tendons

Within the musculoskeletal system tendons have the crucial role to transfer the force exerted by the muscles to the skeleton and, thus, are a critical element for generating movements. As tendon tissue is compliant, the tendon further increase the muscle force potential due to the force-length-velocity relationship and in this way enhance muscle performance (Arampatzis *et al.*, 2009; Magnusson *et al.*, 2007). The non-rigidity of tendons manifests in several physical characteristics. Tendons respond to tensile force with an elongation featuring a pronounced initial increase in length due to collagen crimping at rest. In the subsequent linear region of the force-elongation relation more force is needed to induce the successive lengthening of the collagen fibrils. The slope of the linear region of the force-elongation curve is defined as *tendon stiffness* (Heinemeier, 2011). *In vivo*, human tendon stiffness is determined by dividing the length change of the tendon recorded by ultrasound imaging by the increase of tendon force between 50 and 100% of maximum voluntary muscle contractions (Schulze *et al.*, 2012). The stiffness of a tendon is influenced by its geometrical properties (i.e. cross-sectional area and resting length) and the material properties of the tendon tissue. To assess the material properties of human tendons *in vivo*, the relationship of stress to strain is established by normalizing tendon force to cross-sectional area (obtained from transversal plane magnet resonance images) and the tendon elongation to its resting length. The slope in the linear region of the resulting stress-strain curve is referred to as elastic modulus or *Young's modulus* and is, thus, independent of tendon geometry. The stress at tendon failure is called *ultimate stress* and is highly associated with the material properties of a given tendon. However, due to the viscoelastic nature of the tendon tissue and the associated *creep* deformation, the stress until rupture is substantially lower when tendons are subjected to static stresses (Wang and Ker, 1995).

Functional interaction of muscle and tendon

Within the musculoskeletal system muscle and tendon work as a unit and, thus, the force transmission to the bone and the contraction dynamics of the muscle during movement are directly affected by the mechanical properties of the tendon. A prominent example of this critical interplay is the stretch-shortening cycle. If an active muscle is stretched, the tendon takes over a part of the elongation of the whole muscle-tendon unit. In consequence, the amplitude and velocity of muscle fibre lengthening during the eccentric phase, as well as the shortening during the concentric phase is reduced. This facilitates the force output of the muscle during the contraction due to the force-velocity relationship of muscle fibres. Ishikawa *et al.* (2005) have shown for drop-jumps that the compliance of the Achilles tendon enables the gastrocnemius medialis muscle to work in an isometric-concentric contraction mode despite muscle-tendon unit lengthening. Investigations on running economy demonstrated that more economical runners featured higher levels of Achilles tendon stiffness and muscle strength (Arampatzis *et al.*, 2006). These observations were supported by reports of reductions of oxygen consumption during running after specific training aiming to increase tendon stiffness and muscle of the triceps surae muscle group (Albracht and Arampatzis, 2013.).

The observation that the strain tolerance of tendons is limited and cannot be significantly altered (LaCroix *et al.*, 2013) highlights another crucial aspect of the tendon's mechanical properties regarding the interaction within the muscle-tendon unit. Increases of the muscle's capacity to exert force have to be balanced by a concomitant increase of tendon stiffness to avoid un-physiological tendon strain or tendon failure. Similarly, increases of the tendon's cross-sectional area reduce the tendon stress at a given force and, thus, raise the level of tendon force at stress to failure. However, there is evidence that the transcription of growth factors eliciting adaptational processes of muscle and tendon feature different temporal dynamics (Heinemeier *et al.*, 2011). Further, it has been reported that the mechanical stimuli affecting muscle and tendon adaptation differ as well (Arampatzis *et al.*, 2010). In consequence, the adaptation of the muscle-tendon unit to increased mechanical load might entail the risk of a developing imbalance of muscle strength and loading capacity of the tendon. This assumption is supported by a recent investigation of Couppé *et al.* (2013), demonstrating an association of tendon stress with tendon overuse injury (i.e. patellar tendinopathy). Studies on the Achilles tendon provided evidence that tendinopathy (Arya and Kulig, 2010) and tendon rupture (Hansen *et al.*, 2013) might be related to a mechanical weakening of the tendon.

In conclusion, the mechanical properties of tendons have important implications on the force transmission and coordination between the contractile and the elastic elements within the muscle-tendon unit. Therefore, it is crucial to identify the mechanisms of tendon adaptation and design training interventions to modulate the mechanical properties of tendinous tissue with regard to injury prevention and the efficiency of the muscle-tendon interaction during movement.

Tendon plasticity

Mechanisms of tendon plasticity

As outlined beforehand, tendon properties contribute to various aspects of human locomotor performance (Albracht and Arampatzis, 2013; Arampatzis *et al.*, 2006; Karamanidis *et al.*, 2008; Stafilidis and Arampatzis, 2007) and *vice versa*, locomotion can affect the characteristics of the tendinous tissue (Arampatzis *et al.*, 2007a). The findings of numerous cross-sectional studies of the past years showed that tendon's mechanical and morphological properties are altered in response to specific physical loads (Kongsgaard *et al.*, 2005; Reeves *et al.*, 2003; Rosager *et al.*, 2002), indicating that the tendon is an adaptable biological tissue, which is affected essentially by the exposed daily loading conditions. Comparing inactive control subjects with endurance runners and sprinters, we found a higher tendon stiffness of the triceps surae tendon and aponeurosis and maximal muscle strength only in the sprinters (Figure 1) (Arampatzis *et al.*, 2007a). These results demonstrate a functional adaptation of the tendon in an intensity-dependent manner. An increase in tendon stiffness is achieved by altering either morphological (i.e. cross-sectional area

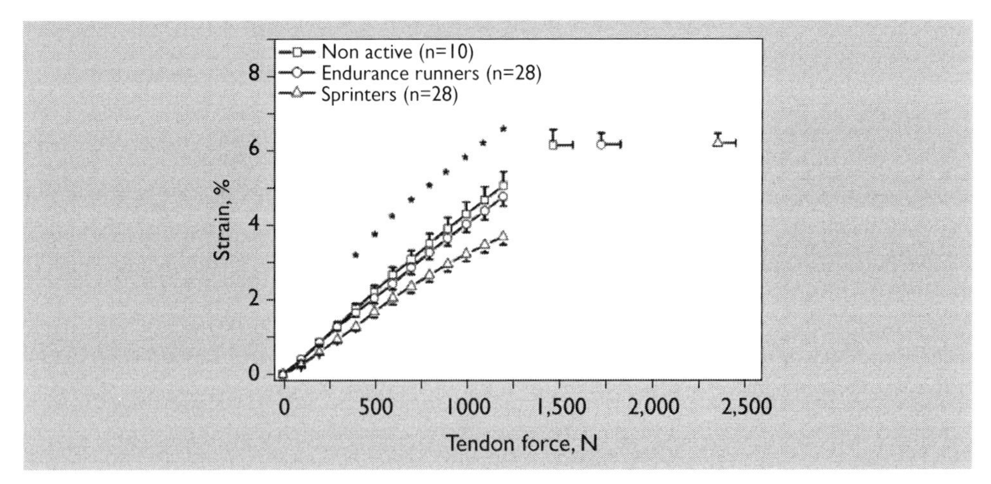

*Figure 1. Strain values at every 100 N and at maximum calculated tendon force of the triceps surae tendon and aponeurosis during maximal voluntary contraction (MVC (mean ± standard error of the mean). * Statistically significant differences between sprinters and the two other groups (P<0.05) (Arampatzis* et al., *2007).*

(CSA)) and/or material properties (i.e. Young's modulus) (Arampatzis *et al.*, 2007b; Kongsgaard *et al.*, 2007; Seynnes *et al.*, 2009). While the latter is considered an early mechanism to increase stiffness, the former is regarded a rather long-term effect of mechanical loading (Heinemeier and Kjaer, 2011; Kjaer *et al.*, 2009).

In contrast to earlier assumptions, research over the past decade provided evidence that tendon tissue is highly metabolically active (Arnoczky *et al.*, 2002; Langberg *et al.*, 2001; Lavagnino and Arnoczky, 2005). Mainly increased collagen synthesis, but also changes in the collagen fibril morphology and collagen cross-link content seems to be responsible for increased tendon stiffness (Heinemeier and Kjaer, 2011; Miller *et al.*, 2005). Within the tendon structure, the physical link of fibroplasts and extracelluar matrix via integrins and other pathways enable the cells to sense and respond to mechanical stimuli (i.e. strain) by regulating the action of collagen stimulating growth factors (Heinemeier and Kjaer, 2011; Kjaer *et al.*, 2009). These so-called mechanotransduction of the external strain to biochemical signals plays the key role in the adaptational response but is, to date, not completely understood (Wang and Thampatty, 2006). Furthermore, in which extend an increased collagen synthesis contributes to either tendon hypertrophy or an alteration of the material properties is also yet unknown (Kjaer *et al.*, 2009).

Tendon adaptation to mechanical loading

Although numerous studies have previously demonstrated a remarkable plasticity of human tendons in response to resistance exercise (Kjaer *et al.*, 2009; Kubo *et al.*, 2001, 2009; Reeves *et al.*, 2003; Seynnes *et al.*, 2009), there is little information about the effect of controlled modulations of specific physical stimuli on the adaptation of mechanical and morphological properties of tendons *in vivo*. However, this specific knowledge is fundamental for the understanding of tendon plasticity. From a mechanobiological point of view, four independent mechanical stimuli can be distinguished: strain magnitude, strain frequency, strain duration and strain rate. In this regard, we investigated the effect of a modulation of these stimuli on the mechanical and morphological properties of the Achilles tendon in controlled exercise interventions (14 weeks, 4 times a week) (Arampatzis *et al.*, 2007b, 2010 and unpublished data). In the first study, one leg was exercised either at low strain magnitude (~2.9%) or high strain magnitude (~4.6%) with the same frequency (3 s loading, 3 s relaxation) and volume by means of isometric plantarflexions at the corresponded intensities of 55% and 90% of the maximum voluntary contraction (MVC), respectively (Arampatzis *et al.*, 2007b). The results showed a decrease in tendon strain at a given tendon force, an increase in tendon elastic modulus (Young's modulus) and a region-specific hypertrophy of the Achilles tendon only in the leg which was exercised at a high strain magnitude (Arampatzis *et al.*, 2007b) (Figure 2). These findings provide evidence for a threshold of a certain strain magnitude *in vivo*, which must be exceeded to evoke adaptational responses of the tendinous tissue. Furthermore, the results indicate that the applied stimulus induced changes in the material as well as morphological properties and, therefore, both adaptational mechanisms were triggered. The protocol with the low strain magnitude did not induce any significant responses and, thus, was considered to not sufficiently exceed the habitual loading to elicit adaptational processes (Arampatzis *et al.*, 2007b) (Figure 2).

To investigate the effect of a modulation of the strain frequency, a second experiment was conducted using the same approach (i.e. low and high strain magnitude), but at higher strain frequency (0.5 Hz, 1

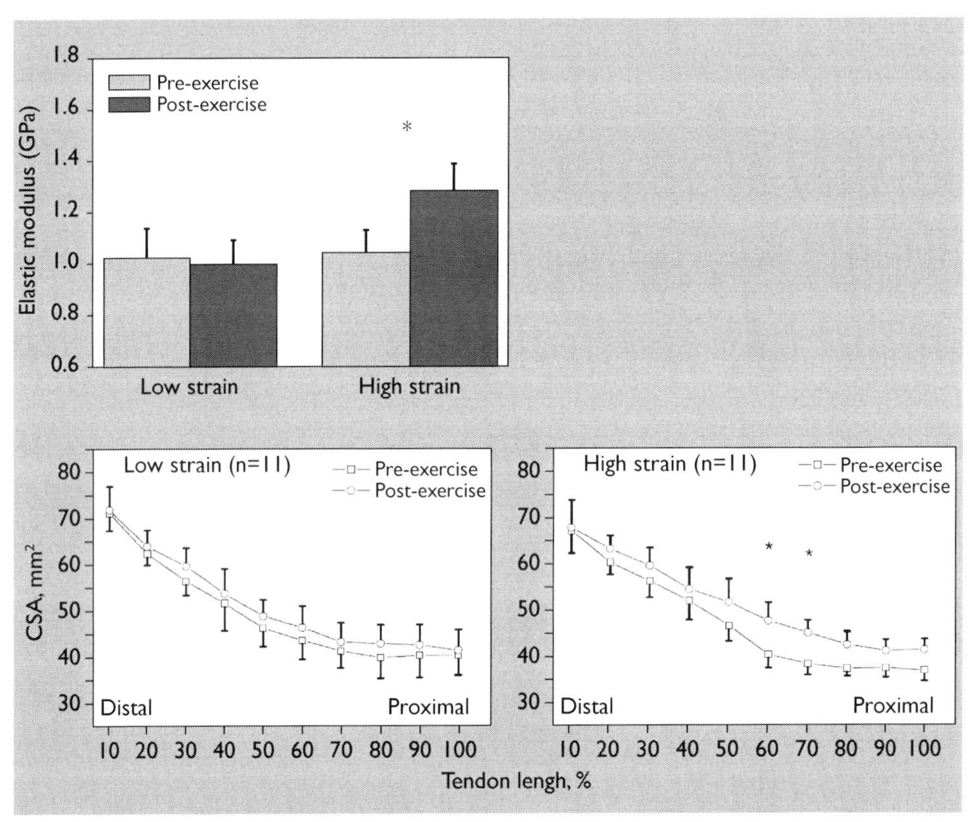

*Figure 2. Achilles tendon elastic modulus (left) and cross-sectional area (CSA) values of the Achilles tendon at every 10% of the tendon length (mid and right) before (pre-exercise) and after (post-exercise) the exercise intervention with low (low strain) and high (high strain) strain magnitudes. * Statistically significant differences between pre- and post-exercise values (P<0.05) (Arampatzis et al., 2007).*

s loading, 1 s relaxation) compared to the previous study (0.17 Hz, 3 s loading, 3 s relaxation). Similarly as in the initial study, only the high strain magnitude protocol induced a change of the mechanical and morphological properties of the Achilles tendon but not the protocol using the low strain magnitude (Arampatzis *et al.*, 2010). Comparing the effectiveness (pre- to post-exercise values) of the high strain magnitude protocols at the different strain frequencies (0.5 versus 0.17 Hz) of both intervention studies, pronounced adaptational responses of the mechanical and morphological properties were observed in the leg exercised at low strain frequency (Figure 3) (Arampatzis *et al.*,

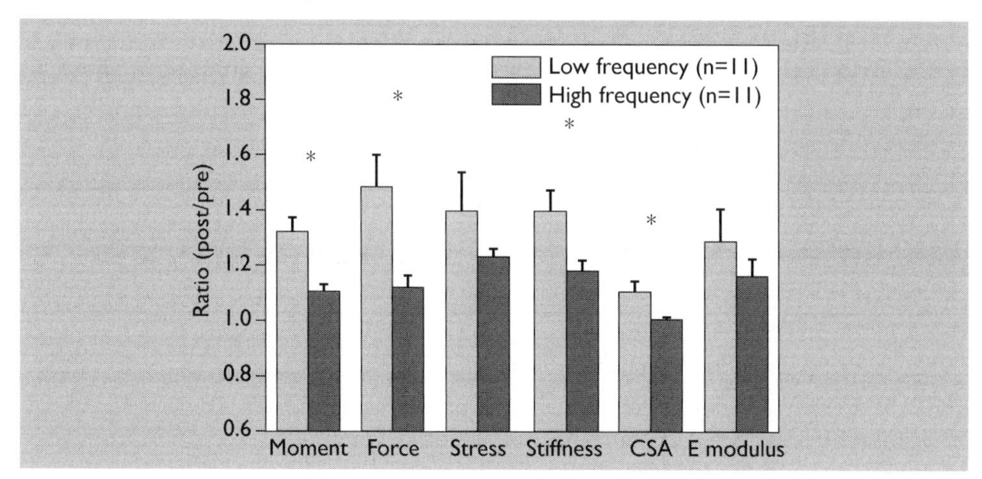

*Figure 3. Ratio (post- to pre-exercise values) of the maximum plantar flexion moment (Moment), maximum calculated tendon force (Force), maximum stress, stiffness of the triceps surae tendon and aponeurosis (Stiffness), average cross-sectional area (CSA) and elastic modulus (E modulus) of the Achilles tendon for the low frequency (0.17 Hz; 3 s loading, 3 s relaxation) and high strain frequency (0.5 Hz; 1 s loading, 1 s relaxation) exercise protocols. * Statistically significant differences between low- and high-frequency exercise protocols (P<0.05) (Arampatzis* et al., *2010).*

2010). Based on these findings, it was concluded that a training using a lower strain frequency with a high strain magnitude is more effective compared to a higher strain frequency.

Just recently, we finished two intervention studies featuring the modulation of the remaining mechanical stimuli: strain rate and strain duration (unpublished data). According to our previous work (Arampatzis *et al.*, 2007b, 2010), the Achilles tendon was again exercised utilizing the same training volume, training period and training sessions per week. However, whereas one leg was trained using a reference protocol with high strain magnitude and low strain frequency (3 s loading, 3 s relaxation; 0.17 Hz), which was set up based on the findings of the previous studies, the other leg was exercised either at a longer strain duration or higher strain rate, respectively. The strain duration was quadruplicated in comparison to the reference protocol and, therefore, a 12 s isometric plantar flexion was performed. To increase the strain rate with respect to the reference protocol, one-legged jumps (72×) featuring higher strain rates due to the short ground contact phases were used as training stimulus. Preliminary results show that the reference protocols and the long strain duration protocol induced similar adaptations of the mechanical and morphological properties of the Achilles tendon (CSA, Young's modulus, stiffness) whereas such responses were not found (CSA, stiffness) in response to the training using the high strain rate.

Taken together, the findings of these interventions suggest that besides the required high strain magnitude a certain time of strain per muscle contraction is necessary to induce adaptational processes, e.g. enhanced collagen synthesis. Since the extracellular matrix features viscoelastic properties, an efficient mechanotransduction of the external load on the cellular level is supposedly time dependent. This could be the reason for the inferior adaptational responses following the intervention using the high strain frequency and high strain rate protocol. In line with this assumption, the similar results of the protocol using the long strain duration and the corresponding reference protocol may indicate that an adequate mechanotransduction occurs within the first seconds (≥3 s).

With respect to practical applications one can conclude from the outlined research that an effective training of the human tendon to affect the mechanical and morphological properties should include strong muscle contractions, which induce a high strain magnitude of the tendon and, therefore, represent adequate adaptational stimuli. The duration of the contraction should be sustained for at least 3 seconds or longer to ensure effective transmission of the external strain on the cellular level. A plyometric training using jumps is not recommended in this regard. These inferences may contribute to the development of efficient training regimens to increase human movement performance and protect the tendon against overuse injury.

References

Albracht, K. and Arampatzis, A., 2013. Exercise-induced changes in triceps surae tendon stiffness and muscle strength affect running economy in humans. European Journal Applied Physiology 113: 1605-1615.

Arampatzis, A., De Monte, G., Karamanidis, K., Morey-Klapsing, G., Stafilidis and S., Brueggemann, G.-P., 2006. Influence of the muscle-tendon unit's mechanical and morphological properties on running economy. Journal of Experimental Biology 209: 3345-3357.

Arampatzis, A., Karamanidis, K. and Albracht, K., 2007b. Adaptational responses of the human Achilles tendon by modulation of the applied cyclic strain magnitude. Journal of Experimental Biology 210: 2743-2753.

Arampatzis, A., Karamanidis, K., Mademli, L. and Albracht, K., 2009. Plasticity of the human tendon to short- and long-term mechanical loading. Exercise and sport sciences reviews 37: 66-72.

Arampatzis, A., Karamanidis, K., Morey-Klapsing, G., De Monte, G. and Stafilidis, S., 2007a. Mechanical properties of the triceps surae tendon and aponeurosis in relation to intensity of sport activity. Journal of Biomechanics 40: 1946-1952.

Arampatzis, A., Peper, A., Bierbaum, S. and Albracht, K., 2010. Plasticity of human Achilles tendon mechanical and morphological properties in response to cyclic strain. Journal of Biomechanics 43: 3073-3079.

Arnoczky, S.P., Tian, T., Lavagnino, M., Gardner, K., Schuler, P. and Morse, P., 2002. Activation of stress-activated protein kinases (SAPK) in tendon cells following cyclic strain: the effects of strain frequency, strain magnitude, and cytosolic calcium. Journal of Orthopedical Research Official Publication Orthopedical Resesearch Society 20: 947-952.

Arya, S. and Kulig, K., 2010. Tendinopathy alters mechanical and material properties of the Achilles tendon. Journal of Applied Physiology 108: 670-675.

Bojsen-Møller, J., Magnusson, S.P., Rasmussen, L.R., Kjaer, M. and Aagaard, P., 2005. Muscle performance during maximal isometric and dynamic contractions is influenced by the stiffness of the tendinous structures. Journal of Applied Physiology 99: 986-994.

Couppé, C., Kongsgaard, M., Aagaard, P., Vinther, A., Boesen, M., Kjaer, M. and Magnusson, S.P., 2013. Differences in tendon properties in elite badminton players with or without patellar tendinopathy. Scandinavian Journal of Medicine & Science in Sports 23: e89-e95.

Finni, T., Peltonen, J., Stenroth, L. and Cronin, N.J., 2013. Viewpoint: On the hysteresis in the human Achillestendon. Journal of Applied Physiology 114: 515-517.

Fletcher, J.R., Esau, S.P. and MacIntosh, B.R., 2010. Changes in tendon stiffness and running economy in highly trained distance runners. European Journal of Applied Physiology 110: 1037-1046.

Hansen, P., Kovanen, V., Hölmich, P., Krogsgaard, M., Hansson, P., Dahl, M., Hald, M., Aagaard, P., Kjaer, M. and Magnusson, S.P., 2013. Micromechanical properties and collagen composition of ruptured human achilles tendon. American Journal of Sports Medicine 41: 437-443.

Heinemeier, K., 2011. *In vivo* investigation of tendon responses to mechanical loading. Journal of Musculoskeletal Neuronal Interaction 11: 115-123.

Heinemeier, K.M., Bjerrum, S.S., Schjerling, P. and Kjaer, M., 2011. Expression of extracellular matrix components and related growth factors in human tendon and muscle after acute exercise. Scandinavian Journal of Medicine & Science in Sports 23: e150-e161.

Ishikawa, M., Niemela, E. and Komi, P.V., 2005. Interaction between fascicle and tendinous tissues in short-contact stretch-shortening cycle exercise with varying eccentric intensities. Journal of Applied Physiology 99: 217-223.

Karamanidis, K., Arampatzis, A. and Mademli, L., 2008. Age-related deficit in dynamic stability control after forward falls is affected by muscle strength and tendon stiffness. Journal of Electromyography and Kinesiology 18: 980-989.

Kjaer, M., Langberg, H., Heinemeier, K., Bayer, M.L., Hansen, M., Holm, L., Doessing, S., Kongsgaard, M., Krogsgaard, M.R. and Magnusson, S.P., 2009. From mechanical loading to collagen synthesis, structural changes and function in human tendon. Scandinavian Journal of Medicine & Science in Sports 19: 500-510.

Kongsgaard, M., Aagaard, P., Kjaer, M. and Magnusson, S.P., 2005. Structural Achilles tendon properties in athletes subjected to different exercise modes and in Achilles tendon rupture patients. Journal of Applied Physiology 99: 1965-1971.

Kongsgaard, M., Reitelseder, S., Pedersen, T.G., Holm, L., Aagaard, P., Kjaer, M. and Magnusson, S.P., 2007. Region specific patellar tendon hypertrophy in humans following resistance training. Acta Physiologica 191: 111-121.

Kubo, K., Ikebukuro, T., Yaeshima, K., Yata, H., Tsunoda, N. and Kanehisa, H., 2009. Effects of static and dynamic training on the stiffness and blood volume of tendon *in vivo*. Journal of Applied Physiology Bethesda Md 1985 106: 412-417.

Kubo, K., Kanehisa, H. and Fukunaga, T., 2001. Effects of different duration isometric contractions on tendon elasticity in human quadriceps muscles. Journal of Physiology 536: 649-655.

LaCroix, A.S., Duenwald-Kuehl, S.E., Lakes, R.S. and Vanderby, R., 2013. Relationship between tendon stiffness and failure: a metaanalysis. Journal of Applied Physiology 115: 43-51.

Langberg, H., Rosendal, L. and Kjaer, M., 2001. Training-induced changes in peritendinous type I collagen turnover determined by microdialysis in humans. Journal of Physiology (London) 534: 297-302.

Lavagnino, M. and Arnoczky, S.P., 2005. *In vitro* alterations in cytoskeletal tensional homeostasis control gene expression in tendon cells. Journal of Orthopedical Research 23: 1211-1218.

Lichtwark, G.A., Bougoulias, K. and Wilson, A.M., 2007. Muscle fascicle and series elastic element length changes along the length of the human gastrocnemius during walking and running. Journal of Biomechanics 40: 157-164.

Lichtwark, G.A., Ker, R.F., Reeves, N.D., Magnusson, S.P., Nordez, A., Arampatzis, A., Vagula, M.C., Cresswell, A.G., Maganaris, C.N., Svensson, R.B., Coupe, C., Hershenhan, A., Eliasson, P., Foure, A., Cornu, C., Morey-Klapsing, G., Mademli, L., Karamanidis, K. and Nelatury, S.R., 2013. Commentaries on Viewpoint: On the hysteresis in the human Achilles tendon. Journal of Applied Physiology 114: 518-520.

Magnusson, S.P., Narici, M.V., Maganaris, C.N. and Kjaer, M., 2007. Human tendon behaviour and adaptation, *in vivo*. Journal of Physiology (London) 586: 71-81.

Miller, B.F., Olesen, J.L., Hansen, M., Døssing, S., Crameri, R.M., Welling, R.J., Langberg, H., Flyvbjerg, A., Kjaer, M., Babraj, J.A., Smith, K. and Rennie, M.J., 2005. Coordinated collagen and muscle protein synthesis in human patella tendon and quadriceps muscle after exercise. Journal of Physiology 567: 1021-1033.

Nigg, B.M. and Herzog, W., 2007. Biomechanics of the musculo-skeletal system, 3rd ed. Wiley, Chichester, UK.

Reeves, N.D., Maganaris, C.N. and Narici, M.V., 2003. Effect of strength training on human patella tendon mechanical properties of older individuals. Journal of Physiology (London) 548: 971-981.

Rosager, S., Aagaard, P., Dyhre-Poulsen, P., Neergaard, K., Kjaer, M., Magnusson and S.P., 2002. Load-displacement properties of the human triceps surae aponeurosis and tendon in runners and non-runners. Scandinavian Journal of Medicine & Science in Sports 12: 90-98.

Schulze, F., Mersmann, F., Bohm, S. and Arampatzis, A., 2012. A wide number of trials is required to achieve acceptable reliability for measurement patellar tendon elongation *in vivo*. Gait & Posture 35: 334-338.

Seynnes, O.R., Erskine, R.M., Maganaris, C.N., Longo, S., Simoneau, E.M., Grosset, J.F. and Narici, M.V., 2009. Training-induced changes in structural and mechanical properties of the patellar tendon are related to muscle hypertrophy but not to strength gains. Journal of Applied Physiology Bethesda Md 1985 107. 523-530.

Stafilidis, S. and Arampatzis, A., 2007. Muscle-tendon unit mechanical and morphological properties and sprint performance. Journal of Sports Science 25: 1035-1046.

Wang, J.H.C. and Thampatty, B.P., 2006. An introductory review of cell mechanobiology. Biomechanics and Modeling in Mechanobiology 5: 1-16.

Wang, X.T. and Ker, R.F., 1995. Creep rupture of wallaby tail tendons. Journal of Experimental Biology 198: 831-845.

Is it possible to train flexor tendons in horses?

Helen Birch
University College London, Stanmore Campus, Brockley Hill, Stanmore, Middlesex, HA7 4LP, United Kingdom; h.birch@ucl.ac.uk

Introduction

The motivation to answer the question of whether tendons are able to adapt to physical training comes primarily from the desire to reduce the incidence of tendon injury. As all those involved with horses know only too well, tendon injuries are notoriously common in competition horses and also in those taking part in less strenuous activities. The flexor tendons in the forelimbs are most at risk with the superficial digital flexor tendon (SDFT) representing more than 75% of tendon injuries in racehorses. A survey of injuries occurring on UK racetracks found that almost one-half (46%) of all limb injuries were due to flexor tendon and/or suspensory ligament (SL) injuries (Williams *et al.*, 2001). Furthermore, tendon injuries that occur on the racetrack represent only the tip of the iceberg; evaluation of a cohort of National Hunt racehorses in training revealed a prevalence of SDFT pathology, detected using ultrasonography, of 24% (Avella *et al.*, 2009). Tendon injuries are one of the most feared injuries as the consequences are severe; repair is slow and full functional recovery is never reached meaning that the horse is more often than not unable to return to the former level of performance. Although many treatments have been advocated, ranging from physical therapies to stem cell implantation, all have a high risk of re-injury. Given the limited ability of current treatments to return a horse with tendinitis to full work without danger of re-injury, prevention of the injury has to be considered as the most appropriate strategy.

Can we make the tendon more robust to physical exercise and less prone to injury?

Traditional training regimes are designed to improve cardiovascular, respiratory and muscular strength and endurance and most often little thought is given to the skeletal system, other than avoiding injury during the training process. Muscle adaptation to physical training is a well-known response and easily observed as muscle hypertrophy. It is also well established, although less obvious, that bone adapts to physical training by changing both mass and architecture. For example, in the serving arms of professional tennis players bone mass can be approximately 30% higher than the non-serving arm. Conversely, reduced mechanical loading, as in bed rest or zero gravity space flight, results in diminished bone mass and resulting weakness. Given that muscle and bone both respond to training by increasing mechanical strength it is not unreasonable to expect that tendon, which forms the link between the two tissues, should also adapt to physical exercise by increasing strength. To date however relatively little is known about the effects of exercise on tendon.

Is their any evidence for tendon adaptation in response to physical training in horses?

A number of training studies have been carried out in horses in an attempt to answer this question. The studies varied in the age of the horses, whether training was treadmill based or over-ground and the length of the training period. A study carried out at the University of Bristol looked at the effect of long-term (18 months) high intensity (HI) training in 18-month-old Thoroughbred horses. The horses ($n = 6$) carried out galloping exercise 3 times a week on a high-speed treadmill and 20 minutes of trotting exercise on days when no galloping was given. The tendons in these horses were compared to an age-matched group of horses ($n = 6$) that carried out only walking exercise (low intensity group (LI)). The simple question of whether tendons undergo adaptive hypertrophy in response to training was addressed by measuring the cross sectional area (CSA) at the end of the study when the horses were 3 years old. Tendon strength was measured by loading tendons to failure in a hydraulic materials testing machine. The CSA of the SDFT in high intensity trained horses was 98 ± 8 mm^2 and not significantly different to that of the low intensity trained horses (105 ± 25 mm^2) (Birch *et al.*, 1999). Furthermore, the mechanical testing showed that there was no difference in the ultimate tensile strength (HI: $13,335 \pm 2,923$ N; LI: $13,335 \pm 2,923$ N) or stiffness (HI: 135 ± 20 kN/strain; LI: 136 ± 17 kN/strain) of the tendons (Birch *et al.*, 2008). It may be that any changes in response to training in this study were masked by individual horse variation, due to relatively small group size. A further similar study was carried out, the only difference being that the horses were trained for 4 months (short term) rather than 18 months as in the previous study. In this study, the CSA of the SDFT was measured using ultrasonography throughout the training period in each horse. The results again showed no change in tendon size with high intensity training (101 ± 9 $mm^{2)}$ compared to low intensity training (99 ± 21 mm^2) (Birch *et al.*, 1999) and no differences in tendon strength and stiffness between groups at the end of the study.

The Bristol studies main focus was on the SDFT as this tendon is the most common site of injury in racehorses and therefore of particular interest. The equine SDFT however is an 'energy-storing' tendon and one of the most extreme examples of a tendon with this specialized spring-like function, which may have some bearing on the outcome. The spring-like function enables the tendon to store elastic strain energy and then return the energy thereby reducing the energetic cost of locomotion. The stiffness of an energy-storing tendon is finely tuned to allow the most efficient energy return. An increase in the CSA of an energy-storing tendon would result in increased stiffness of the structure and this would be detrimental to tendon function. The anatomically opposed common digital flexor tendon (CDET) in the horse functions to extend the distal part of the limb, playing a role in limb placement. Tendons such as the equine CDET are known as 'positional' tendons. Unlike energy-storing tendons, positional tendons are required to have high stiffness for efficient function so that minimal extension occurs, ensuring that muscle shortening results in joint movement. Coincidentally the equine CDET rarely gets injured. In the long term and short term Bristol training studies the CSA of the CDET was also measured. Following long-term training, as in the SDFT, there was no difference in CDET CSA between high (31 ± 3 mm^2) and low (32 ± 2 mm^2) intensity trained horses (Birch *et al.*, 1999). Following short-term training however the high intensity trained group of horses had a significantly larger CDET (29 ± 3 mm^2) than the low intensity trained group (25 ± 2 mm^2). Interestingly, the CSA of the high intensity trained group was not significantly different to both groups in the long-term training study where horses were a year older. This finding suggests that the CDET grows in size between 2 and 3 years of age and that training can increase the rate of growth.

The SDFT appears to reach maturity at an earlier age so a training effect on growth could not be seen in these studies (Birch *et al.*, 1999).

The results of these studies prompted further training studies to determine whether training in very young horses (foals) can result in an increase in the CSA of the SDFT. A study carried out in Japan trained foals from 2 months of age using galloping exercise on a treadmill. The CSA of the SDFT was followed ultrasonographyically throughout the 13-month training program. The results showed an increased rate of growth of the SDFT in the treadmill trained foals compared to age-matched non-trained foals; however at the end of the study there was no significant difference in SDFT size between groups (Kasashima *et al.*, 2002). These results suggest that there is a window of opportunity to influence tendon properties during maturation.

Hypertrophy of the tendon is perhaps the simplest aspect to consider, however training may result in a change in the material properties of the tendon tissue. Tendon is composed primarily of water, the fibrous protein collagen and a non-collagenous component consisting of proteoglycans and glycoproteins. The collagen component has a hierarchical arrangement from collagen molecules to fibrils, fibres and finally fascicles which group together to form the whole tendon. Changes in the amount and/or organization of these components will change the mechanical properties of the tendon material thereby changing overall properties of the tendon without a change in size. In the Bristol long term training study the water content and collagen content of the SDFT did not differ between high and low intensity trained groups (Birch *et al.*, 2008). The collagen however showed a difference in organization in the central zone of the SDFT with an increased population of small diameter fibrils in high intensity trained horses (mass-average fibril diameter (MAFD): 105.3 ± 4.3 nm) compared to the low intensity trained group (MAFD: 131.7 ± 4.9 nm) (Patterson-Kane *et al.*, 1997). In addition, in the same region of the tendon the high-intensity trained group showed significantly reduced glycosaminoglycan content; a component that is thought to play a role in controlling collagen fibril diameters. Although these changes might be expected to result in a difference in mechanical properties of the tissue no differences were detected in ultimate stress or elastic modulus when tendons were mechanically tested (Birch *et al.*, 2008). The differences seen in SDFT matrix composition and organization following long term high intensity training were not observed in the short term study, suggesting that 4 months of exercise is not sufficient time to influence these properties.

One of the important points to consider with respect to the changes observed following long term training are whether these represent adaptive changes to improve tendon properties or whether they represent damage. Smaller diameter collagen fibrils may result from synthesis of new collagen or break down of existing collagen fibrils. The SDFT from the long-term study showed no signs of immature collagen crosslinks or younger less fluorescent collagen suggesting that breakdown of old collagen fibrils had occurred (Birch *et al.*, 2008). The mechanism for this breakdown and the impact on mechanical properties are not clear, as overall mechanical properties were not significantly different between groups.

It has become apparent that measuring the mechanical properties of the whole tendon is too basic an approach. For example, we know very well from epidemiological studies that tendon injuries are more common with increasing age (Ely *et al.*, 2009), but testing whole equine flexor and extensor tendons shows no difference in strength or stiffness with increasing age (Thorpe *et al.*, 2013b). The mechanical properties of the whole structure are achieved through a combination of the properties at each hierarchical level. Furthermore, to consider only ultimate strength and stiffness may miss the subtler, but very important properties of tendon, particularly with respect to specialized energy storing tendons. The SDFT, as an energy-storing tendon, is subjected to relatively high strains of around 16% at the gallop, a loading rate of approximately 200%/sec and a high number of repetitions. The positional CDET, although subjected to the same number of loading and unloading cycles, experiences much lower strains (about 3%) at lower rates of loading (12.5%/sec). It is important that the SDFT is both an efficient spring and fatigue resistant under these extreme conditions of loading.

Our more recent work has started to build an understanding of how specific mechanical requirements are achieved by studying the sub levels of structure in the complex multi-composite hierarchical tendon. Fascicles, which group together to form the whole tendon, are surrounded by a connective tissue or inter-fascicular matrix known as the endotenon. Fascicles can be carefully dissected from the tendon and mechanically tested in isolation or bound to another fascicle to give the properties of the inter-fascicular matrix. Although studies of whole tendons have shown that the equine SDFT fails at a higher strain than the CDET (Batson *et al.*, 2003), conversely, fascicles from the SDFT failed at a lower strain than those from the CDET (Thorpe *et al.*, 2013b). In the SDFT however the inter-fascicular matrix is less stiff, enabling greater fascicle sliding and greater extension. Furthermore the fascicles themselves differ in their extension mechanism; fascicle extension in the CDET is dominated by fibre sliding whereas fascicles in the SDFT rely on unwinding of a helical structure (Thorpe *et al.*, 2013a). This helical structure may also be responsible for the greater recovery following loading and unloading, lower hysteresis and greater fatigue resistance of SDFT fascicles compared to fascicles from the CDET.

In view of this work, it is now apparent that tendon mechanical properties should be studied at the fascicle and fibre level in future training studies and that hysteresis and fatigue measurements should also be made. Furthermore, our recent work presents the exciting prospects that it may, in addition to reducing injuries, be possible to improve performance. For example, adaptation of the interfascicular matrix to allow more efficient return of energy would reduce the energetic cost of locomotion by reducing muscular effort required.

Conclusion

In conclusion, there is still much to be learnt with regards to tendon response to training. However, we can say with some certainty, that although the SDFT of older horses is able to undergo high strains it may be more susceptible to fatigue damage due to age related changes. In young horses short-term high-intensity training does not appear to be damaging however longer-term training may result in tendon micro-damage. Training at a very young age is not detrimental to tendon and furthermore may take advantage of a window of opportunity for tendon adaptation. Continued effort into understanding the biology and mechanics of tendon will improve our ability to design training programs to reduce tendon injuries and may also provide the exciting possibility to improve performance through appropriate changes to tendon structure.

References

Avella, C.S., Ely, E.R., Verheyen, K.L., Price, J.S., Wood, J.L. and Smith, R.K., 2009. Ultrasonographic assessment of the superficial digital flexor tendons of National Hunt racehorses in training over two racing seasons. Equine Vet J 41: 449-454.

Batson, E.L., Paramour, R.J., Smith, T.J., Birch, H.L., Patterson-Kane, J.C. and Goodship, A.E., 2003. Are the material properties and matrix composition of equine flexor and extensor tendons determined by their functions? Equine Vet J 35: 314-318.

Birch, H.L., McLaughlin, L., Smith, R.K. and Goodship, A.E., 1999. Treadmill exercise-induced tendon hypertrophy: assessment of tendons with different mechanical functions. Equine Vet J Suppl 30: 222-226.

Birch, H.L., Wilson, A.M. and Goodship, A.E., 2008. Physical activity: does long-term, high-intensity exercise in horses result in tendon degeneration? J Appl Physiol 105: 1927-1933.

Ely, E.R., Avella, C.S., Price, J.S., Smith, R.K., Wood, J.L. and Verheyen, K.L., 2009. Descriptive epidemiology of fracture, tendon and suspensory ligament injuries in National Hunt racehorses in training. Equine Vet J 41: 372-378.

Kasashima, Y., Smith, R.K., Birch, H.L., Takahashi, T., Kusano, K. and Goodship, A.E., 2002. Exercise-induced tendon hypertrophy: cross-sectional area changes during growth are influenced by exercise. Equine Vet J Suppl: 264-268.

Patterson-Kane, J.C., Wilson, A.M., Firth, E.C., Parry, D.A. and Goodship, A.E., 1997. Comparison of collagen fibril populations in the superficial digital flexor tendons of exercised and nonexercised thoroughbreds. Equine Vet J 29: 121-125.

Thorpe, C.T., Klemt, C., Riley, G.P., Birch, H.L., Clegg, P.D. and Screen, H.R., 2013a. Helical sub-structures in energy-storing tendons provide a possible mechanism for efficient energy storage and return. Acta Biomater 9: 7948-7956.

Thorpe, C.T., Udeze, C.P., Birch, H.L., Clegg, P.D. and Screen, H.R., 2013b. Capacity for sliding between tendon fascicles decreases with ageing in injury prone equine tendons: a possible mechanism for age-related tendinopathy? Eur Cell Mater 25: 48-60.

Williams, R.B., Harkins, L.S., Hammond, C.J. and Wood, J.L., 2001. Racehorse injuries, clinical problems and fatalities recorded on British racecourses from flat racing and National Hunt racing during 1996, 1997 and 1998. Equine Vet J 33: 478-486.

Equine carpal osteoarthritis and thoracic limb function: effects of aquatic rehabilitation

Melissa R. King[1], Kevin K. Haussler[1], Christopher E. Kawcak[1], C. Wayne McIlwraith[1], Raoul F. Reiser II[2], David D. Frisbie[2] and Natasha M. Werpy[3]
[1]Gail Holmes Equine Orthopaedic Research Center, Colorado State University, 1678 Campus Delivery, Fort Collins, CO 80532-1678, USA; [2]Department of Health and Exercise Science, Colorado State University, 220 Moby B Complex, Fort Collins, CO 80523-1582, USA; [3]Department of Small Animal Clinical Sciences, University of Florida, P.O. Box 100126, Gainesville, FL 32610-0126, USA; melissa.king@colostate.edu

Take home message

Aquatic therapy for the management of carpal osteoarthritis demonstrates both disease-modifying and measurable clinical improvements.

Introduction

Osteoarthritis (OA) is one of the most debilitating musculoskeletal disorders among equine athletes (Peloso *et al.*, 1994). It is a progressive disease characterized by joint pain, inflammation, synovial effusion, limited range of motion, and a progressive deterioration of articular cartilage (McIlwraith and Vachon, 1988). Unremitting joint pain and inflammation often cause adaptive muscle guarding and altered weight bearing to protect the affected limb from further discomfort and injury (Weishaupt, 2008). In humans, compensatory changes in posture and movement exacerbate the initial joint injury, which cause further alterations in limb biomechanics and contribute to the progression of OA (Astephen *et al.*, 2008). Similar compensatory mechanisms such as altered muscle activation patterns, increased joint stiffness, and a redistribution of limb loading, are likely to also occur in horses.

Physical rehabilitation has become an effective treatment option for primary musculoskeletal injuries and for reducing or limiting harmful compensatory gait abnormalities in humans (Hurley, 1997).

Rehabilitation programs that address OA and musculoskeletal injuries often incorporate some form of aquatic exercise. Exercising in water provides an effective medium for increasing joint mobility, increasing muscle activation, promoting normal motor patterns, and reducing the incidence of secondary musculoskeletal injuries (Prins and Cutner, 1999). Underwater treadmill exercise has become an increasingly popular therapy for the rehabilitation of equine musculoskeletal injuries; unfortunately, there is no scientific evaluation of its effectiveness for the treatment of OA. This project was established to investigate the physiologic, biomechanical, and histologic effects of aquatic therapy on diminishing the progression of OA within the equine middle carpal joint. Results from this study will provide an objective assessment of the pathologic characteristics associated with OA and the potential clinical and disease-modifying effects allied with aquatic therapy.

Materials and methods

Horses

Sixteen skeletally mature horses, aged 2 to 4 years (mean $\pm$ SD body weight, 385 ± 40 were included in the study. The Colorado State University Institutional Animal Care and Use Committee approved the study protocol.

Experimental design and induction of osteoarthritis

An osteochondral fragment (OCF) was created in 1 randomly selected middle carpal joint of each horse. An 8-mm-wide fragment was generated with an 8-mm curved osteotome directed perpendicular to the articular cartilage surface of the radial carpal bone at the level of the medial synovial plica (Frisbie *et al.*, 2002).

Exercise

Beginning on day 15, all horses were exercised on a high-speed overground treadmill 5 days each week, until the end of the study to promote the development of OA. Each day, the horses were trotted at 4.4 m/s for 2 minutes, galloped at 8.8 m/s for 2 minutes, and trotted again at 4.4 m/s as part of a standard exercise protocol used to aid in the induction and progression of carpal joint OA.

Treatment groups

The aquatic exercise group was exposed to underwater treadmill exercise starting on day 15. The underwater treadmill protocol consisted of exercise at a brisk walk (2.1 m/s), once a day, for 5 days. The water level in the underwater treadmill was maintained at the point of the shoulder for the duration of the study, which reduced weight bearing by approximately 60% (McClintock *et al.*, 1987). At weekly intervals, the duration of underwater treadmill exercise was increased by 5 minutes, until a maximum of 20 min/session was reached. Horses then continued to be exercised for 20 minutes once a day, 5 days a week, for the remainder of the 10-week study (i.e. 8 weeks of exercise). The control group was exercised on an overground treadmill (without water) in a manner similar to that of the underwater treadmill protocol for the intervention group (i.e. same speed, frequency, and duration of exercise), also starting at day 15. The overground treadmill exercise undertaken by the control group was designed to simulate conventional hand walking and light exercise used for rehabilitation after arthroscopic surgery.

Data collection

Displacement of the center of mass (COM) of each horse's body was determined from center of pressure (COP) measurements recorded with 2 strain-gauge-based force platforms (60×90 cm) mounted in series in a concrete base. Postural sway data were collected from each horse at 4 time points during the study: prior to induction of the osteochondral fragment (day -7), after induction of the osteochondral fragment (day 14), 4 weeks after initiating treadmill exercise (day 42), and at study conclusion (day 70). Horses were made to stand stationary on the force platforms under 3 stance conditions: normal square stance, base-narrow placement of the thoracic limbs, and removal of visual cues (blindfolded) during a normal square stance. For each stance condition, each horse was required to stand quietly for 3 consecutive, 10-second trials. The mean of the 3 trial results in each condition was calculated and used for analysis.

Ground reactions forces (GRF), thoracic limb kinematics, and electromyographic (EMG) activity were recorded simultaneously from each horse during the above mentioned time points. For data collection, horses were trotted in hand at a self-selected, uniform velocity (2.8 to 3.4 m/s) and trials were not accepted if the velocity was >10% of the average baseline for each horse. Forward velocity was measured using a series of 5 infrared emitters and corresponding reflective sensors placed 2 m apart. The initial ground contact and toe-off events for each step per 10-s trial were identified with a biaxial accelerometer adhered to the dorsolateral hoof wall of both front hooves. The on-off hoof events were used to determine EMG timing of select thoracic limb muscles during the stance and swing phases over a minimum of 2 strides. Kinetic, kinematic and EMG temporal variables were averaged across three trials and normalized to stride duration.

Weekly evaluations included clinical assessments of lameness, response to carpal flexion, and thoracic limb passive joint range of motion. Horses were euthanized 70 days after osteochondral fragmentation and gross pathologic and histologic examinations of cartilage and synovial membrane specimens from the middle carpal joint were performed.

Statistical analysis

Statistical software was used to evaluate data using an ANOVA or ANCOVA framework depending on the presence or absence of a covariate, respectively. ANOVA tables were used to determine significant ($P<0.05$) main effects and interactions between main-effect variables.

Results

Craniocaudal postural sway

Craniocaudal sway differed significantly ($P=0.04$) depending on the stance conditions; the blindfolded horses had the largest amplitudes of craniocaudal sway, compared with the base-narrow and normal square stance conditions (Table 1). Craniocaudal sway was significantly ($P<0.001$) influenced by the presence or absence of aquatic exercise. Horses exercised in the underwater treadmill had significantly decreased craniocaudal sway, compared with that of the control group (Table 2). When specific individual comparisons were conducted, craniocaudal sway in the blindfolded normal square

Table 1. Mean ± standard error of the mean normalized postural sway variables obtained from all 16 horses when they were in a normal square stance position, a base-narrow stance position, and a blindfolded normal square stance position, controlling for the effects of time and treatment group.

COP variable	**Stance position**		
	Normal	**Base-narrow**	**Blindfolded**
Craniocaudal sway (%)	1.3±0.1[b]	1.4±0.1[b]	1.6±0.1[a]
Mediolateral sway (%)	4.8±0.5[b]	6.5±0.5[a]	6.0±0.5[a]
COP area (%)	69.0±17.7[b]	112.0±17.7[a]	126.0±17.7[a]
COP velocity (mm/s)	13.9±1.1[b]	14.8±1.1[a]	16.1±1.1[a]
COP radius (mm)	4.6±0.3	4.5±0.3	4.7±0.3

[a,b] Within a row, different superscript letters indicate significant (P<0.05) differences between the stance positions.

stance position was significantly decreased at days 42 (P=0.004) and 70 (P=0.03) in the aquatic exercise group, compared with findings in the control groups.

Mediolateral postural sway

Mediolateral sway differed significantly (P=0.01) depending on the stance position. Significantly increased amplitudes of mediolateral sway were evident in the base-narrow and blindfolded normal square stance positions, compared with that in the normal square stance position (Table 1). Horses undergoing underwater treadmill exercise had significantly (P< 0.001) reduced mediolateral sway, compared with that of control horses (Table 2). Horses exercised on the underwater treadmill had significantly (P=0.02) decreased mediolateral sway when blindfolded in the normal square stance position on day 42 (4.8 ± 0.7%), compared with that of the horses exercised on the overground treadmill (7.1 ± 0.7%).

Thoracic limb loading patterns

The magnitude of the thoracic limb craniocaudal COP movement toward or away from the limb with the surgically created osteochondral fragment in the carpal joint was significantly (P=0.02) influenced

Table 2. Mean ± standard error of the mean postural sway variables obtained from the 2 groups of horses at 28 and 56 days after commencement of treadmill exercise (i.e. days 42 and 70 after surgical creation of an osteochondral fragment in one randomly selected carpal joint), controlling for the effect of stance position and study day.

COP variable	**Treatment**	
	Control	**UWT**
Craniocaudal sway (%)	1.7±0.1[a]	1.1±0.1[b]
Mediolateral sway (%)	6.6±0.3[a]	4.4±0.3[b]
COP area (%)	135.2±11.0[a]	56.4±11.0[b]
COP velocity (mm/s)	15.1±0.8[a]	12.5±0.8[b]
COP radius (mm)	5.5±0.2[a]	3.6±0.2[b]

[a,b] Within a row, different superscript letters indicate significant (P<0.05) differences between the treatment groups.

by the presence of the osteochondral fragment, depending upon the stance position and applied treatment. When individual comparisons were conducted, the craniocaudal COP location shifted significantly (P<0.001) toward the unaltered thoracic limb in the blindfolded normal square stance position within the control group (2.2±0.1%), compared with findings for the limb with the surgically created osteochondral fragment (1.5±0.1%). In addition, the blindfolded normal square stance position in the control group resulted in a significantly (P<0.001) greater shift in the location of the craniocaudal COP toward the unaltered thoracic limb (2.2±0.1%), compared with findings for the unaltered thoracic limb in horses exercised on the underwater treadmill (1.3±0.1%). Similarly, the craniocaudal COP displacement during the base-narrow stance position had a significantly (P=0.007) greater shift toward the unaltered thoracic limb in the control group (1.7±0.1%), compared with findings for the unaltered thoracic limb in horses exercised on the underwater treadmill (1.2±0.1%). Under both stance conditions, horses in the control group had a significant shift of the craniocaudal COP away from the limb with the surgically created osteochondral fragment, thereby unloading the injured and presumably painful joint.

Ground reaction forces

Peak vertical GRF's (PFz) differed significantly ($P=0.02$) between OCF and unaltered thoracic limbs depending on whether the horse had underwater treadmill exercise or simulated hand walking (overground treadmill). Individual comparisons within the control group revealed that OCF limbs had a decreased PFz ($P=0.007$), compared to unaltered limbs. However, there were no significant differences between the OCF and unaltered limbs within the aquatic therapy group.

Electromyography

Onset of muscle activity was significantly ($P=0.05$) delayed within the OCF limb, compared to the unaltered limb (Figure 1). Ulnaris lateralis (UL) onset of muscle activity was also significantly ($P=0.02$) influenced by the induction of an OCF and the applied treatment. Within the control group the OCF limb had a significantly delayed onset of UL muscle activity ($91 \pm 1\%$; $P=0.004$), compared to the

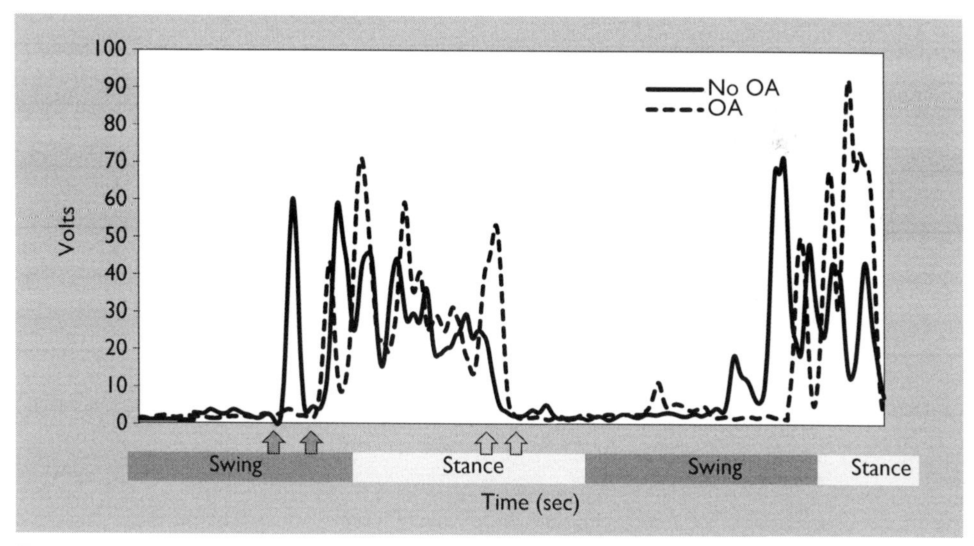

Figure 1. Representative ulnaris lateralis muscle activation profile from the OCF (dashed line) and unaltered limbs (solid line). The solid black arrows demonstrate the significant difference in the onset of muscle activity within the OCF ulnaris lateralis compared to the ulnaris lateralis muscle onset of activity within the unaltered limb. The open arrows demonstrate termination of muscle activity within the ulnaris lateralis.

contralateral muscle (88 ± 1%). However, there were no significant differences between the OCF and unaltered limbs within the aquatic therapy group.

Goniometry

OCF significantly ($P=0.01$) decreased carpal flexion angles throughout the study period. OCF carpal flexion angles were significantly ($P=0.02$) improved in aquatic therapy horses (31.0 ± 1.0 degrees), compared to the control OCF carpus (34.0 ± 1.0 degrees). Significant improvements in carpal flexion angles within the underwater treadmill group began on day 21 and continued throughout the remainder of the study. At study conclusion there was no significant difference between the aquatic therapy OCF and unaltered passive carpal flexion angles; the use of underwater treadmill exercise returned carpal joint range of motion to baseline values.

Histologic examination

Significantly increased synovial membrane intimal hyperplasia occurred within the OCF joint (score 1.5 ± 0.2; $P=0.009$), compared to contralateral unaltered joints (0.6 ± 0.2). In addition, a significant ($P=0.05$) treatment effect was noted with decreased intimal hyperplasia in unaltered joints (0.1 ± 0.3) exercised in the underwater treadmill, compared to the control unaltered joints (1.1 ± 0.3). Underwater treadmill exercise demonstrated a disease modifying effect as it reduces the degree of synovial membrane inflammation.

Discussion

The results of this study provide the first evidence that aquatic therapy for the management of carpal OA demonstrates both disease-modifying and measurable clinical improvements. Underwater treadmill exercise was able to re-establish baseline levels of carpal flexion, returning the carpal joint to full range of motion. In addition, horses exercised in the underwater treadmill demonstrated evenly distributed thoracic limb axial loading, symmetrical timing of select thoracic limb musculature, and significant improvements in static balance control under various stance conditions. The improvement in clinical signs of OA in the aquatic therapy group was further supported by evidence of disease-modifying effects at the histologic level. Underwater treadmill exercise reduced joint capsule fibrosis and decreased the degree of inflammatory infiltrate present in the synovial membrane.

The increased resistance and buoyancy inherent in aquatic exercise minimizes joint instability and weight bearing stresses applied to limbs (Evans *et al.*, 1978). Humans with osteoarthritis who are involved in aquatic treatment programs often have a significant reduction in pain, increase in muscle strength, and improvement in motor control (Giaquinto *et al.*, 2007). Neuromotor control of on-off muscle timing is crucial for producing coordinated movements and maintaining joint stability. The induction of middle carpal joint OA in the current study produced asynchronous muscle activation patterns, which ultimately may have influenced the magnitude and rate of limb loading, impaired proprioception, and altered active joint range of motion. These neuromuscular alterations may be the result of joint pain and inflammation, altering afferent signalling from the joint mechanoreceptors and thus influencing the ability to coordinate muscle activity. The application of aquatic therapy demonstrated an ability to maintain symmetrical timing of select carpal extensor muscles. Exercising in the underwater treadmill maintained timely neuromotor control between the thoracic limbs contributing to coordinated muscle activity, symmetrical limb loading, and functional joint stability. Conversely, the delayed muscle activation within the control OCF limbs may have contributed to an imbalance in muscle timing leading to incoordination and unequal attenuation of mechanical stresses applied across the middle carpal joint.

Overall, the precise mechanisms by which aquatic therapy positively influenced clinical signs and demonstrated disease-modifying effects is unclear. Nevertheless, results from this study indicate that underwater treadmill exercise is a potentially viable therapeutic option in managing OA in horses, which is fundamental to providing evidence-based support for equine aquatic treatment.

References

Astephen, J.L., Deluzio, K.J., Caldwell, G.E., Dunbar, M.J. and Hubley-Kozey, C.L., 2008. Gait and neuromuscular pattern changes are associated with differences in knee osteoarthritis severity levels. J Biomech 41: 868-876.

Evans, B., Cureton, K. and Purvis, J., 1978. Metabolic and circulatory responses to walking and jogging in water. Res Q 49: 442-449.

Frisbie, D., Ghivizzani, C., Robbins, P., Evans, C. and McIlwraith, C.W., 2002. Treatment of experimental equine osteoarthritis by *in vivo* delivery of the equine interleukin-1 receptor antagonist gene. Gene Ther 9: 12-20.

Giaquinto, S., Ciotola, E., Margutti, F. and Valentini, F., 2007. Gait during hydrokinesitherapy following total hip arthroplasty. Disability and Rehabilitation 29: 743-749.

Hurley, M.V., 1997. The effects of joint damage on muscle function, proprioception and rehabilitation. Manual Therapy 2: 11-17.

McClintock, S.A., Hutchins, D.R. and Brownlow, M.A., 1987. Determination of weight reduction in horses in flotation tanks. Equine Vet J 19: 70-71.

McIlwraith, C. and Vachon, A., 1988. Review of pathogenesis and treatment of degenerative joint disease. Equine Veterinary Journal Supplement 20: 3-11.

Peloso, J.G., Mundy, G.D. and Cohen, N.D., 1994. Prevalence of, and factors associated with, musculoskeletal racing injuries of Thoroughbreds. J Am Vet Med Assoc 204: 620-626.

Prins, J. and Cutner, D., 1999. Aquatic therapy in the rehabilitation of athletic injuries. Clin Sports Med 18: 447-460.

Weishaupt, M., 2008. Adaptation strategies of horses with lameness. Vet Clin North Am Equine Pract 21: 79-100.

Tendon rehabilitation in human athletes

Kirsten Legerlotz
School of Biological Sciences, University of East Anglia, Norwich Research Park, Norwich NR4 7TJ, United Kingdom; k.legerlotz@uea.ac.uk

Take home message

Tendinopathies, chronic tendon disorders characterized by pain and functional impairment, are a common problem particularly in elite and recreational athletes, as well as in the sedentary population. It has been shown that exercise or mechanical loading plays a role, which is why overuse is suspected to initiate tendinopathies. The exact mechanisms are still poorly understood, which makes the treatment problematic. Although a variety of treatment options are available, most of them focus solely on symptom relief, and the evidence for their effectiveness is often poor. However, exercise treatment has been relatively well investigated, has been shown to work in the majority of cases and is considered the gold standard.

Introduction

The adaptation of connective tissues to exercise is often equalized with an increase in performance, which is in turn equalized with an increase in strength, cross sectional area and the change of composition and mechanical properties. In muscle, those changes are often clearly visible and easily measurable. In tendon however, adaptation is usually less obvious. While some studies find a greater cross sectional area in exercised tendons (Kongsgaard *et al.*, 2005; Rosager *et al.*, 2002), others don't (Hansen *et al.*, 2003; Huang *et al.*, 2004; Legerlotz *et al.*, 2007), and while some find the mechanical properties changing (Arampatzis *et al.*, 2007; Kubo *et al.*, 2002), others do not (Karamanidis and Arampatzis, 2006). The reason for the apparently limited adaptation capacity might be rooted in both the low metabolic activity of tendon tissue as well as the functional requirements. Tendon tissue has a very slow turn over time of about 200 years (Thorpe *et al.*, 2010) and the cells within the tissue appear to be dominantly dormant (Heinemeier *et al.*, 2013). This implies that once a tendon is fully developed upon maturity the tendon matrix is able to withstand a lifetime of loading without much need for adaptation. The adaptation capacity might also be limited by tendon function: on the one hand the tendon has to transmit forces from muscle to bone, in which case it would be advantageous to be thick and stiff, while on the other hand the tendon also acts as spring to reduce energy expenditure, in which case it would be advantageous to be thin, long and elastic. This means that there is not much room for big changes, although high loads experienced over several years as in elite sports might tip the balance slightly to the thick and stiff side. However, even if exercise might not lead to measurable compositional or biomechanical changes, the tendon cells are required to maintain this equilibrium. If this equilibrium is disturbed, e.g. by excessive loading, tendinopathies might develop.

Pathophysiology of tendinopathies

The term tendinopathy compasses any painful condition occurring within or around the tendon, characterized by localized activity related pain, tenderness to palpation, edema and functional impairment (Skjong *et al.*, 2012). Traditionally this condition has been called tendinitis, but since there was no histopathological evidence for inflammation, the general term tendinopathy was adopted, to encompass both degradation and inflammation as possible mechanisms (Riley, 2004). Tendinopathy is associated with a variety of morphological, histopathological, biochemical and molecular changes. Morphologically it is associated with an increase in tendon cross sectional area, decreased fibril diameter, loss of fibre organization, infiltration of blood vessels, thickened tendon sheath and hypoechoic areas (Khan *et al.*, 1999; Riley, 2005). Histological slides similarly show disorganized fibres and in addition lipid and calcific deposits, increased proteoglycan content, an increase in cell density and cell rounding (Astrom and Rausing, 1995; Chard *et al.*, 1994; Riley, 2005). Biochemical changes reflecting the condition are a decreased content in total collagen, an accumulation in type III collagen, an altered cross-linking pattern, increased glycosaminoglycan, aggrecan and biglycan content (Riley *et al.*, 1994a,b, 1996, 2001). These changes in composition are associated with an increase in gene expression of certain matrix proteins (e.g. collagen type I and III, aggrecan, biglycan and tenascin C), cytokines and signalling factors (e.g. TGF-b, COX2, IGF1 and VEGF) and degrading enzymes (e.g. MMP1, MMP2 and ADAM12) while a range of other degrading enzymes decrease in gene expression (e.g. MMP3, MMP10 and ADAMTS5) (Corps *et al.*, 2004, 2006; Jones *et al.*, 2006). However, there is no uniform molecular signature of tendinopathy, as e.g. IL6 and COX2 increase in Achilles tendinopathy while they do not change with posterior tibialis tendinopathy (Legerlotz *et al.*, 2012).

A variety of intrinsic factors (e.g. age, joint laxity, anatomical variants, muscle weakness, gender, body weight, systemic disease) and extrinsic factors (occupation, shoes, temperature, running surface, training regime) have been discussed as plausible contributors to the development of tendinopathies (Kannus *et al.*, 2002; Riley, 2004). Only, there is no simple cause and effect chain and it remains unclear while some people develop the syndrome being subjected to comparatively normal levels of loading while some elite athletes subjecting their tendons for a long duration to enormous levels of high loading never develop any symptoms. However, loading or exercise remains the strongest factor correlating with the development of tendinopathies. On this basis the micro-trauma-theory has been developed to explain the pathophysiology of tendinopathies (Kannus *et al.*, 2002; Riley, 2004). According to the micro-trauma-theory single collagen fibres will rupture when the tendon is strained beyond physiological levels of strain. Normal movement is assumed not to lead to more than 4% strain, which should be far below the failure threshold of a whole healthy tendon. If the tendon is repeatedly strained beyond this threshold, the micro-ruptures will accumulate, which will eventually lead to regional structural changes weakening the tendon, even resulting in the rupture of the whole tendon.

According to Cook and Purdam (2009) three different stages of tendinopathy should be distinguished:

1. Reactive tendinopathy: caused by a rapid increase in loading or trauma, leading to thickening/swelling of the tendon and pain, as a reversible adaptation to overload.
2. Tendon disrepair: caused by continuous excessive loading, leading to a change in tendon structure through matrix breakdown and neovascularization
3. Degenerative tendinopathy: following on the disrepair stage and caused by chronic overloading leading to irreversible changes associated with advanced matrix breakdown and disorganized collagen structure.

Treatment options

A variety of treatment options are available to treat tendinopathies. However, the majority of these procedures are only supported by limited evidence. Since the pathophysiological mechanisms are unclear most treatments focus on symptom relief.

Exercise treatment

The concept is to use heavy loading (eccentric, eccentric-concentric or heavy slow resistance training) as a stimulus to induce tendon cell activity and matrix restructuring, utilizing the self-healing capacities of the tendon. It has been well documented that this type of rehabilitation program leads to pain relief, reduces neovascularisation and improves tendon structure. Although the exact modalities (types of exercise, duration and intensities, should athletes be withdrawn from training) are still discussed, this procedure is generally well accepted and so far considered the gold-standard. It has to be kept in mind though, that it might not be suitable in the acute reactive stage of tendinopathy (Cook and Purdam, 2009). Also, following the exercise program will require time and effort, and a poor compliance will most likely lead to a poor outcome (Saithna *et al.*, 2012). In contrast to the most commonly used eccentric training protocol developed by Alfredson *et al.* (1998), the heavy slow resistance training (Kongsgaard *et al.*, 2009) requires less time, though access to a gym and a good technique are essential, which might limit it to athletes at a higher level.

Corticosteroid injections

Since there are no histopathological signs of inflammation in the tendinopathic tendon core and inflammation has been ruled out to play a major role in tendinopathy, it is difficult to justify the use of corticosteroids. However, corticosteroid injections are now aimed at the inflammatory response of the surrounding tissue and are still widely used (Coombes *et al.*, 2010). They are indeed effective with regards to pain relief (Kongsgaard *et al.*, 2009), but there is no long term benefit and this treatment is not affecting the underlying cause. It has also be considered, that corticosteroids might have detrimental effects on tendon structure. They have been shown to inhibit collagen synthesis (Wong *et al.*, 2004) and to affect the mechanical properties of the tendon (Mikolyzk *et al.*, 2009), which might increase the risk of tendon rupture.

Nonsteroidal anti-inflammatory drugs

Assuming that tendinopathy is a non-inflammatory condition the concept behind this popular treatment option seems unclear. They are prescribed for pain-relief, although there is little evidence supporting this treatment option (Almekinders and Temple, 1998). As the collagen synthesis after running exercise was inhibited with use of nonsteroidal anti-inflammatory drugs (NSAIDs), they are thought to possibly affect the adaptation to exercise negatively and should thus be used with caution (Christensen *et al.*, 2011).

Platelet-rich plasma

The idea behind this treatment option, to augment tendon healing by injection of beneficial biological factors contained in the plasma, is convincing, but the evidence is conflicting. A double-blind, randomized, placebo-controlled trial on the clinical use of platelet-rich plasma injection did not show any improvement compared to the placebo (De Vos *et al.*, 2010). In animal studies a positive effect of platelet-rich plasma on surgically induced tendon injuries has been found (Bosch *et al.*, 2010, 2011), but it is questionable whether a surgically induced lesion of a healthy tendon is an adequate model for tendinopathy.

Stem cell therapy

Mesenchymal stem cells are injected at the injury site to promote tendon healing. The stem cells are thought to differentiate into tenocytes, to replace the lost or damaged cells and to initiate repair mechanisms in the injured region. Equine studies have shown an improved histological tissue appearance and a reduced re-injury rate with stem cell injection (Godwin *et al.*, 2012; Pacini *et al.*, 2007). This form of treatment seems promising and no adverse side-effects have been reported, however, the current evidence is sparse and no data on humans are available. Furthermore, the fate of the injected cells is unclear, and it has yet to be established if they actually stay and/or survive at the site of injury.

Sclerosing agents

Since blood vessel accompanying nerves are thought to contribute to the pain in tendinopathy, this therapy aims at destroying neovessels and their accompanying nerves by injection of caustic agents. The limited evidence shows that this form of treatment effectively reduces pain, neovessels and tendon swelling (Alfredson and Ohberg, 2005; Lind *et al.*, 2006; Ohberg and Alfredson, 2003). However, it purely focuses on symptoms, while the function of the neovessels is yet to be determined.

Prolotherapy

The concept behind prolotherapy is to inject large volumes of fluid with the aim to disrupt neovessels and to reinitiate inflammatory processes kick starting the healing process. Considering that prolotherapy has been developed in the 1930s, the evidence for its effectiveness in tendinopathy is surprisingly limited (Crisp *et al.*, 2008) and good quality studies are rare.

Topical nitroglycerin patches

Application of topical nitroglycerin patches on the skin near the site of injury aim to increase the nitric oxide concentration in the tissue, which is supposed to reduce pain and to improve the tendon matrix by induction of fibroblast differentiation and collagen synthesis. The mechanism of action has yet to be proven and the evidence regarding its effectiveness is limited. In patients suffering from Achilles tendinopathy a reduction in tendon pain and tenderness compared to a placebo has been shown (Paoloni and Murrell, 2007; Paoloni *et al.*, 2004;). However, headaches can occur as possible side effect (Gambito *et al.*, 2010).

Shock-wave therapy

The administration of a series of shock-waves to a painful tendon aims to disrupt neovascularization and to increase tenocyte proliferation. This is supposed to reduce pain and to initiate a micro-trauma related healing response, although a proof of this concept is lacking. A few studies described shock-wave therapy as effective tool in the management of tendinopathies (Rompe *et al.*, 2008, 2009). However, a randomized placebo-controlled trial showed no improvement with shock-wave therapy, but suggests an increased risk of tendon rupture in older patients (Costa *et al.*, 2005).

Surgical debridement

The surgery aims to excise fibrotic adhesions, to disrupt neovessels and to promote wound repair, thereby leading to a relief of symptoms and a return to function. It has to be kept in mind that this is no quick fix, but a highly invasive procedure, bearing the risk of complications and the need for rehabilitation. Success rate and long term outcome are not clear, since both seem to depend on the quality of the study ('the poorer the methodology the higher the success rate' (Coleman *et al.*, 2000). A randomized controlled trial did not show any superiority of surgical intervention compared with eccentric strength training (Bahr *et al.*, 2006).

Future directions

Although there are a variety of treatment options available, there is only limited evidence of the success of most of them. More good quality randomized-placebo controlled trials are needed to test treatment methods on their effectiveness. Basic research into the initiation and progression of tendinopathy might aid in developing successful treatment methods. To test those treatment methods it would be advantageous if a valid tendinopathy-animal-model could be established. The success rate of treatment options might be enhanced if the treatment would be tailored to the individual characteristics of the patient as well as the stage and site of tendinopathy. To date exercise treatment is considered the gold standard, however, exercise treatment protocols still need to be specified, and they could be adapted to treat other forms of tendinopathy (e.g. hamstrings, supraspinatus) and other populations (e.g. equine).

Conclusion

It might be confusing to choose the adequate treatment option from the variety of available ones. However, one might be guided by the principle not to do harm, and to avoid concepts that have not been proven to work or which have known side-effects:

- *Staging.* First of all it seems important to determine the stage of the tendinopathy to tailor the treatment adequately (Cook and Purdam, 2009)
- *Load management.* Since tendinopathy is a load induced tendon problem, load should be managed sensibly, e.g. irritable exercises, compression, high intensities for a long duration should be avoided (Cook and Purdam, 2012). To choose alternative exercise (e.g. to replace running by swimming or vice versa) and to plan rest might support the recovery process.
- *Pain management.* Pain is the most dominant symptom in tendinopathy, leading to discomfort and the inability to exercise. Thus pain management has an important role. Isometric exercises can reduce pain (Naugle *et al.*, 2012), the short term use of pain killers/NSAIDs in the reactive stage, and sclerosing agents and nitroglycerin patches in the disrepair stage would also be an option.
- *Strength rehabilitation.* Both the tendinopathy itself as well as first line treatment could have reduced tendon strength. Secondly, to avoid a relapse it is advisable to only gradually increase training

Table 1. Examples of established exercise treatment protocols.

Study	**Tendon**	**Exercise type**	**Treatment period**	**Treatment frequency**	**Exercise prescription**
Alfredson *et al.*, 1998	Achilles tendon	eccentric	12 weeks	twice daily	Two types of unilateral heel drops: with straight leg and with knee bent. Non-affected leg used for upward component. 3 sets of 15 repetitions. Successively increasing load by adding weight.
Kongsgaard *et al.*, 2009	Patellar tendon	heavy slow resistance	12 weeks	three times per week	3 bilateral exercises: squat, leg press and hack squat to 90° flexion. 4 sets with 2-3 min rest. Increasing load from 15 repetition maximum (RM) in week 1 to 6 RM in week 9-12.
Kongsgaard *et al.*, 2009	Patellar tendon	eccentric	12 weeks	twice daily	Eccentric unilateral squats on a 25% decline board, upward component on unaffected leg. 3 sets of 15 repetitions, 2 min rest between sets. Successively increasing load by adding weight.

intensity and duration. Established eccentric (Alfredson *et al.*, 1998) or heavy resistance (Kongsgaard *et al.*, 2009) tendon rehabilitation protocols can help to recover strength and function (Table 1), but should not be applied in the acute reactive stage.

References

Alfredson, H. and Ohberg, L., 2005. Neovascularisation in chronic painful patellar tendinosis--promising results after sclerosing neovessels outside the tendon challenge the need for surgery. Knee Surg Sports Traumatol Arthrosc 13: 74-80.

Alfredson, H., Pietila, T., Jonsson, P. and Lorentzon, R., 1998. Heavy-load eccentric calf muscle training for the treatment of chronic Achilles tendinosis. Am J Sports Med 26: 360-366.

Almekinders, L.C. and Temple, J.D., 1998. Etiology, diagnosis, and treatment of tendonitis: an analysis of the literature. Med Sci Sports Exerc 30: 1183-1190.

Arampatzis, A., Karamanidis, K., Morey-Klapsing, G., De Monte, G. and Stafilidis, S., 2007. Mechanical properties of the triceps surae tendon and aponeurosis in relation to intensity of sport activity. J Biomech 40: 1946-1952.

Astrom, M. and Rausing, A., 1995. Chronic Achilles tendinopathy. A survey of surgical and histopathologic findings. Clin Orthop Relat Res: 151-164.

Bahr, R., Fossan, B., Loken, S. and Engebretsen, L., 2006. Surgical treatment compared with eccentric training for patellar tendinopathy (Jumper's knee). A randomized, controlled trial. J Bone Joint Surg Am 88: 1689-1698.

Bosch, G., Moleman, M., Barneveld, A., Van Weeren, P.R. and Van Schie, H.T., 2011. The effect of platelet-rich plasma on the neovascularization of surgically created equine superficial digital flexor tendon lesions. Scand J Med Sci Sports 21: 554-561.

Bosch, G., Van Schie, H.T., De Groot, M.W., Cadby, J.A., Van de Lest, C.H., Barneveld, A. and Van Weeren, P.R., 2010. Effects of platelet-rich plasma on the quality of repair of mechanically induced core lesions in equine superficial digital flexor tendons: A placebo-controlled experimental study. J Orthop Res 28: 211-217.

Chard, M.D., Cawston, T.E., Riley, G.P., Gresham, G.A. and Hazleman, B.L., 1994. Rotator cuff degeneration and lateral epicondylitis: a comparative histological study. Ann Rheum Dis 53: 30-34.

Christensen, B., Dandanell, S., Kjaer, M. and Langberg, H., 2011. Effect of anti-inflammatory medication on the running-induced rise in patella tendon collagen synthesis in humans. J Appl Physiol 110: 137-141.

Coleman, B.D., Khan, K.M., Maffulli, N., Cook, J.L. and Wark, J.D., 2000. Studies of surgical outcome after patellar tendinopathy: clinical significance of methodological deficiencies and guidelines for future studies. Victorian Institute of Sport Tendon Study Group. Scand J Med Sci Sports 10: 2-11.

Cook, J.L. and Purdam, C.R., 2009. Is tendon pathology a continuum? A pathology model to explain the clinical presentation of load-induced tendinopathy. Br J Sports Med 43: 409-416.

Cook, J.L. and Purdam, C.R., 2012. Is compressive load a factor in the development of tendinopathy? Br J Sports Med 46: 163-168.

Coombes, B.K., Bisset, L. and Vicenzino, B., 2010. Efficacy and safety of corticosteroid injections and other injections for management of tendinopathy: a systematic review of randomised controlled trials. Lancet 376: 1751-1767.

Corps, A.N., Robinson, A.H., Movin, T., Costa, M.L., Hazleman, B.L. and Riley, G.P., 2006. Increased expression of aggrecan and biglycan mRNA in Achilles tendinopathy. Rheumatology 45: 291-294.

Corps, A.N., Robinson, A.H., Movin, T., Costa, M.L., Ireland, D.C., Hazleman, B.L. and Riley, G.P., 2004. Versican splice variant messenger RNA expression in normal human Achilles tendon and tendinopathies. Rheumatology 43: 969-972.

Costa, M.L., Shepstone, L., Donell, S.T. and Thomas, T.L., 2005. Shock wave therapy for chronic Achilles tendon pain: a randomized placebo-controlled trial. Clin Orthop Relat Res 440: 199-204.

Crisp, T., Khan, F., Padhiar, N., Morrissey, D., King, J., Jalan, R., Maffulli, N. and Frcr, O.C., 2008. High volume ultrasound guided injections at the interface between the patellar tendon and Hoffa's body are effective in chronic patellar tendinopathy: A pilot study. Disabil Rehabil 30: 1625-1634.

De Vos, R.J., Weir, A., Van Schie, H.T., Bierma-Zeinstra, S.M., Verhaar, J.A., Weinans, H. and Tol, J.L., 2010. Platelet-rich plasma injection for chronic Achilles tendinopathy: a randomized controlled trial. JAMA 303: 144-149.

Gambito, E.D., Gonzalez-Suarez, C.B., Oquinena, T.I. and Agbayani, R.B., 2010. Evidence on the effectiveness of topical nitroglycerin in the treatment of tendinopathies: a systematic review and meta-analysis. Arch Phys Med Rehabil 91: 1291-1305.

Godwin, E.E., Young, N.J., Dudhia, J., Beamish, I.C. and Smith, R.K., 2012. Implantation of bone marrow-derived mesenchymal stem cells demonstrates improved outcome in horses with overstrain injury of the superficial digital flexor tendon. Equine Vet J 44: 25-32.

Hansen, P., Aagaard, P., Kjaer, M., Larsson, B. and Magnusson, S.P., 2003. Effect of habitual running on human Achilles tendon load-deformation properties and cross-sectional area. J Appl Physiol 95: 2375-2380.

Heinemeier, K.M., Schjerling, P., Heinemeier, J., Magnusson, S.P. and Kjaer, M., 2013. Lack of tissue renewal in human adult Achilles tendon is revealed by nuclear bomb (14)C. FASEB J 27: 2074-2079.

Huang, T.F., Perry, S.M. and Soslowsky, L.J., 2004. The effect of overuse activity on Achilles tendon in an animal model: a biomechanical study. Ann Biomed Eng 32: 336-341.

Jones, G.C., Corps, A.N., Pennington, C.J., Clark, I.M., Edwards, D.R., Bradley, M.M., Hazleman, B.L. and Riley, G.P., 2006. Expression profiling of metalloproteinases and tissue inhibitors of metalloproteinases in normal and degenerate human achilles tendon. Arthritis Rheum 54: 832-842.

Kannus, P., Paavola, M., Paakkala, T., Parkkari, J., Jarvinen, T. and Jarvinen, M., 2002. [Pathophysiology of overuse tendon injury]. Radiologe 42: 766-770.

Karamanidis, K. and Arampatzis, A., 2006. Mechanical and morphological properties of human quadriceps femoris and triceps surae muscle-tendon unit in relation to aging and running. J Biomech 39: 406-417.

Khan, K.M., Cook, J.L., Bonar, F., Harcourt, P. and Astrom, M., 1999. Histopathology of common tendinopathies. Update and implications for clinical management. Sports Med 27: 393-408.

Kongsgaard, M., Aagaard, P., Kjaer, M. and Magnusson, S.P., 2005. Structural Achilles tendon properties in athletes subjected to different exercise modes and in Achilles tendon rupture patients. J Appl Physiol 99: 1965-1971.

Kongsgaard, M., Kovanen, V., Aagaard, P., Doessing, S., Hansen, P., Laursen, A.H., Kaldau, N.C., Kjaer, M. and Magnusson, S.P., 2009. Corticosteroid injections, eccentric decline squat training and heavy slow resistance training in patellar tendinopathy. Scand J Med Sci Sports 19: 790-802.

Kubo, K., Kanehisa, H. and Fukunaga, T., 2002. Effects of resistance and stretching training programmes on the viscoelastic properties of human tendon structures *in vivo*. J Physiol 538: 219-226.

Legerlotz, K., Jones, E.R., Screen, H.R. and Riley, G.P., 2012. Increased expression of IL-6 family members in tendon pathology. Rheumatology 51: 1161-1165.

Legerlotz, K., Schjerling, P., Langberg, H., Bruggemann, G.P. and Niehoff, A., 2007. The effect of running, strength, and vibration strength training on the mechanical, morphological, and biochemical properties of the Achilles tendon in rats. J Appl Physiol 102: 564-572.

Lind, B., Ohberg, L. and Alfredson, H., 2006. Sclerosing polidocanol injections in mid-portion Achilles tendinosis: remaining good clinical results and decreased tendon thickness at 2-year follow-up. Knee Surg Sports Traumatol Arthrosc 14: 1327-1332.

Mikolyzk, D.K., Wei, A.S., Tonino, P., Marra, G., Williams, D.A., Himes, R.D., Wezeman, F.H. and Callaci, J.J., 2009. Effect of corticosteroids on the biomechanical strength of rat rotator cuff tendon. J Bone Joint Surg Am 91: 1172-1180.

Naugle, K.M., Fillingim, R.B. and Riley, J.L., 3rd, 2012. A meta-analytic review of the hypoalgesic effects of exercise. J Pain 13: 1139-1150.

Ohberg, L. and Alfredson, H., 2003. Sclerosing therapy in chronic Achilles tendon insertional pain-results of a pilot study. Knee Surg Sports Traumatol Arthrosc 11: 339-343.

Pacini, S., Spinabella, S., Trombi, L., Fazzi, R., Galimberti, S., Dini, F., Carlucci, F. and Petrini, M., 2007. Suspension of bone marrow-derived undifferentiated mesenchymal stromal cells for repair of superficial digital flexor tendon in race horses. Tissue Eng 13: 2949-2955.

Paoloni, J.A., Appleyard, R.C., Nelson, J. and Murrell, G.A., 2004. Topical glyceryl trinitrate treatment of chronic noninsertional achilles tendinopathy. A randomized, double-blind, placebo-controlled trial. J Bone Joint Surg Am 86-A: 916-922.

Paoloni, J.A. and Murrell, G.A., 2007. Three-year followup study of topical glyceryl trinitrate treatment of chronic noninsertional Achilles tendinopathy. Foot Ankle Int 28: 1064-1068.

Riley, G.P., 2004. The pathogenesis of tendinopathy. A molecular perspective. Rheumatology 43: 131-142.

Riley, G.P., 2005. Gene expression and matrix turnover in overused and damaged tendons. Scand J Med Sci Sports 15: 241-251.

Riley, G.P., Goddard, M.J. and Hazleman, B.L., 2001. Histopathological assessment and pathological significance of matrix degeneration in supraspinatus tendons. Rheumatology 40: 229-230.

Riley, G.P., Harrall, R.L., Cawston, T.E., Hazleman, B.L. and Mackie, E.J., 1996. Tenascin-C and human tendon degeneration. Am J Pathol 149: 933-943.

Riley, G.P., Harrall, R.L., Constant, C.R., Chard, M.D., Cawston, T.E. and Hazleman, B.L., 1994a. Glycosaminoglycans of human rotator cuff tendons: changes with age and in chronic rotator cuff tendinitis. Ann Rheum Dis 53: 367-376.

Riley, G.P., Harrall, R.L., Constant, C.R., Chard, M.D., Cawston, T.E. and Hazleman, B.L., 1994b. Tendon degeneration and chronic shoulder pain: changes in the collagen composition of the human rotator cuff tendons in rotator cuff tendinitis. Ann Rheum Dis 53: 359-366.

Rompe, J.D., Furia, J. and Maffulli, N., 2008. Eccentric loading compared with shock wave treatment for chronic insertional achilles tendinopathy. A randomized, controlled trial. J Bone Joint Surg Am 90: 52-61.

Rompe, J.D., Furia, J. and Maffulli, N., 2009. Eccentric loading versus eccentric loading plus shock-wave treatment for midportion achilles tendinopathy: a randomized controlled trial. Am J Sports Med 37: 463-470.

Rosager, S., Aagaard, P., Dyhre-Poulsen, P., Neergaard, K., Kjaer, M. and Magnusson, S.P., 2002. Load-displacement properties of the human triceps surae aponeurosis and tendon in runners and non-runners. Scand J Med Sci Sports 12: 90-98.

Saithna, A., Gogna, R., Baraza, N., Modi, C. and Spencer, S., 2012. Eccentric exercise protocols for patella tendinopathy: should we really be withdrawing athletes from sport? A Systematic Review. Open Orthop J 6: 553-557.

Skjong, C.C., Meininger, A.K. and Ho, S.S., 2012. Tendinopathy treatment: where is the evidence? Clin Sports Med 31: 329-350.

Thorpe, C.T., Streeter, I., Pinchbeck, G.L., Goodship, A.E., Clegg, P.D. and Birch, H.L., 2010. Aspartic acid racemization and collagen degradation markers reveal an accumulation of damage in tendon collagen that is enhanced with aging. J Biol Chem 285: 15674-15681.

Wong, M.W., Tang, Y.N., Fu, S.C., Lee, K.M. and Chan, K.M., 2004. Triamcinolone suppresses human tenocyte cellular activity and collagen synthesis. Clin Orthop Relat Res: 277-281.

Applying functional electrical stimulation in the rehabilitation of muscle and tendons in horses

Sheila Schils
EquiNew, LLC, N8139 900th St, River Falls, WI 54022, USA;
sbschils@equinew.com

Take home message

FES is a specific class of electrotherapy that has been developed for use in equine rehabilitation. Treatments with FES have shown promise in reducing muscle spasms or atrophy, strengthening muscles and reeducating muscle memory to improve function and symmetry after injury or surgery. In addition, FES has been used in a limited number of cases to improve tendon and ligament healing in the distal limb. FES has been used extensively in human rehabilitation and the potential for use in horses is developing.

Introduction

The use of modalities to aid in rehabilitation protocols is a developing science and there are many tools equine practitioners can use to assist in the implementation of a rehabilitation plan. An understanding of these tools helps the practitioner to decide which modalities should be used, and when. One of these emerging tools for rehabilitation, which will be discussed in this paper, is called functional electrical stimulation (FES).

FES is a specific class of electrotherapy and is distinctly different from other electrotherapy devices such as transcutaneous electrical nerve stimulator (TENS), galvanic and high-voltage pulsed-current (HVPC) stimulators (Schils, 2009). The term FES is sometimes used interchangeably with neuromuscular electrical stimulation (NMES) systems, and while FES is a type of NMES, this exact exchange of names is not accurate. The American Physical Therapy Association outlines the designations of the classes of electrotherapy devices (Alon *et al.*, 2005), but manufacturers do not always carefully follow these designations. Care must be taken when evaluating an electrotherapy device, because some systems may be labelled as a different class from what their parameters are.

FES produces controlled muscular contractions through the use of a specific electrical current that has been generated by software. The electrical signal produced by FES creates an action potential in the peripheral nerve, which then activates muscle contractions in the related muscle tissue (Rattay *et al.*, 2003). The FES signal is designed so that it is almost indistinguishable to those produced by the body's own nervous system (Stackhouse, 2008). Contractions of muscles by FES at higher intensities produces coordinated limb or body movements generating joint movement. Therefore, controlled movement can be obtained by FES not only by the muscles, but also by the associated tendons and ligaments. The movement obtained using FES is almost identical to the movement observed in the functional coordination of muscles needed to perform a task (Stackhouse, 2008), therefore giving the therapy its name. In comparison, other nerve and muscle stimulators do not produce true muscle contractions and obtain only a tremor or a twitch in the muscle that is being stimulated. Joint movement can be obtained by these systems with higher amplitudes, however the voltage needed is typically 10 times higher than required by FES. In addition, joint movements from these types of electrotherapy devices are rough, quick and non-functional.

The correct FES signal is a balanced waveform that does not allow for an accumulation of charge (a galvanic action). Due to the design of the FES system, 'the delivered charge is extracted out of the targeted tissue at the end of every single stimulation pulse' (Masani and Popovic, 2011). This feature is an important aspect when looking at the long-term safety of FES, especially in cases of continual use such as for bladder control or neuroprosthesis. Further evaluation of the safety of the use of FES, for up to 10-years, has focused on fragile, denervated muscle. In these studies, a decrease in damaged fibres and an increase in functional fibres were found with long-term use of FES (Carraro *et al.*, 2005).

Differences do exist in how the muscle fibre types respond to electrical stimulation, when compared to the response elicited by the brain.

In the normal physiological activation of slow- and fast-twitch fibres, fast-twitch fibres are only activated when quickness and speed are obtained. However, during FES treatments, both slow- and fast-twitch fibre recruitment occurs at the same time (Gregory and Bickel, 2005). This aspect can be very beneficial for many rehabilitation protocols because these fast-twitch muscle fibres may not be accessed for several months. FES can be used to activate all fibre types helping to avoid fibre atrophy during the rehabilitation period, therefore allowing for faster and greater strength gains (Harrelson *et al.*, 1998). In addition, as a further aid to healing, FES has been shown to increase the size of myofibres and cause regeneration of new myofibres (Kern *et al.*, 2004).

Discussing the transfer of the application of FES from human rehabilitation into equine therapy is the focus of this paper. This paper will outline the use of FES in human rehabilitation and conversely how this technology is being implemented in equine rehabilitation protocols.

Functional electrical stimulation use in human rehabilitation

Several decades ago FES was first used in the rehabilitation of spinal cord injury patients to generate muscle movement to prevent atrophy. Today, FES has been shown to be effective for multiple purposes including the treatment of both spastic and flaccid muscle and to restore grasping and reaching functions (Kawashima *et al.*, 2008; Thrasher *et al.*, 2008). Studies in rats that evaluated the neuroplasticity of reinnervation has shown that FES can delay muscle atrophy by producing better nerve conduction and higher muscle weights (Lim and Han, 2010) and can restore muscle size, and functional and histochemical properties when compared to no stimulation (Marqueste *et al.*, 2006). Additional human studies have shown the ability of FES to reverse muscle atrophy for denervated muscle tissue to obtain standing and walking in spinal cord injury patients (Gallien *et al.*, 1995; Graupe and Kohn, 1998; Graupe *et al.*, 2008; Mushahwar *et al.*, 2007; Yarkony *et al.*,1990). Other research on humans has shown that FES can prevent and even reverse atrophy of chronically denervated muscles when evaluated by muscle biopsies and knee extension torque (Kern *et al.*, 2002; Kern *et al.*, 2005; Kern *et al.*, 2008).

FES has also been utilized to suppress spasticity in many studies. FES was shown to successfully decrease muscle spasticity related to cerebral palsy (Johnston and Wainwright, 2011) and multiple sclerosis (Krause *et al.*, 2007). Even in the cases of strong flexor spasticity in the hands of hemiplegic stroke patients, stimulation of the extensors by FES was able to obtain hand opening. However, it was interesting to note that extensor stimulation did not reduce flexor activity as hypothesized, probably due to the generation of the stretch reflex (Hines, 1994). Spastic leg musculature was significantly reduced when FES cycling was implemented with spinal cord injury patients, resulting in an increase in isometric torque and less fatigue (Szecsi and Schiller, 2009). In other related studies, abnormal joint stiffness associated with spastic muscle, decreased up to 53% when FES was used (Mirbagheri *et al.*, 2002). In addition, a decrease in quadriceps spasticity, an increase in strength and an increase in stride length were found with the use of FES in partial spinal cord injury patients (Granat *et al.*, 1993). Even long-term spasticity in hemiplegic patients showed a significant improvement in strength when FES was utilized (Stefanovska *et al.*, 1989).

Reeducation of muscle memory has also been shown to be a result of FES. Studies of FES spinal cord injury patients found improved muscle movement even when FES was not being applied (Popovic *et al.*, 2009). An evaluation of the use of FES for gait rehabilitation after stroke, showed that retraining strategies, which included FES, were more effective than retraining alone. Near infrared spectroscopy (fNIRS) was used to determine the neuroplasticity of the cortex, which occurred during retraining with FES (Belda *et al.*, 2001). In addition, FES was used to show improved motor functional recovery and improved range of motion in hemiplegic patients when compared to controls (Wang *et al.*, 2002). Another interesting study of 10 patients with chronic facial nerve paralysis showed improvement in facial muscle movement with electrotherapy when other forms of treatment were non-effective (Hyvarinen *et al.*, 2008).

Cardiovascular exercise can be obtained for spinal cord injury patients using FES to pedal a bicycle. Improvements were observed in muscle endurance, speed, and strength and increases in aerobic metabolism and endurance were seen, although the changes were not more than would be obtained with voluntary exercise (Arnold *et al.*, 1992; Pollack *et al.*, 1989). Other human studies found a significant increase in heart rate and an improvement in blood flow (Faghri *et al.*, 2001), and an increased respiratory rate during FES cycling (Jacobs *et al.*, 2003) for spinal cord injury patients, which improved their overall conditioning and health.

Functional electrical stimulation use in equine rehabilitation

FES has been utilized in equine rehabilitation for almost 20 years, however the number of practitioners using FES is small. The FES technology for equine practice was modified from equipment used for humans, and treatment protocols specific to the horse were developed. FES has been shown to be a useful modality, in a limited number of horses, for the reduction of muscle spasms and atrophy (Schils, 2010), and muscle wasting (Schils, 2012).

The majority of the FES applications on horses has focused on treatments of epaxial and deep muscle spasms and atrophy. Ultrasound video taken during FES stimulation at T17-18 has shown that the signal can penetrate to the psoas muscle.

A pad, similar to a saddle pad, is used to hold 6 electrodes (3 on each side) in place so that the signal is symmetrical when the pad is used over the spine. The intensity of the FES signal is increased slowly until small contractions are felt or seen. The higher the voltage the deeper the signal will penetrate. Typically the first contractions are seen in top line treatments at approximately 3-5 volts. The voltage is increased as long as the horse is comfortable and at 5-9 volts spinal flexion or joint movement is usually observed. The degree of movement is dependent upon the purpose of the treatment and the comfort of the horse. In certain situations, such as acute tendon tears, the voltage is controlled so that only the cells are stimulated and no movement is obtained. Compliance to the treatment is excellent. No sedation is required and sedation is actually contraindicated. This is due to the fact that the horse's reaction to the increase in voltage is important to determine how much movement should be asked for.

The response of the muscle to the stimulation, observed in the degree and type of contractions under each electrode, is noted.

Horses, depending on their specific muscular or skeletal problems, will respond differently to the stimulus. Some horses will show slow, steady contractions, followed by a slow, steady relaxation mimicking the signal of the FES system. In contrast, other horses will show distinct fasciculations with no clear pattern or relaxation phase in response to the stimulus. The joint movement during the FES treatments in some horses will be smooth, while other horses will show rough, jerky movement. The association between a smooth, steady contraction/relaxation cycle, that mimics the FES signal, to healthy well-functioning muscle seems to be prevalent.

When the electrodes are positioned so that the signal crosses the spine, bilateral, symmetrical functional movement can be obtained. When the pad is placed over the sacroiliac, the horse sometimes show a twist to the pelvic rotation rather than symmetrical caudal/cranial movement. If the muscle physiology of the horse is distinctly asymmetrical, the movement obtained through FES stimulation seems to reflect that. Therefore, the practitioner can observe the dynamic movement of the muscles and associated joints, or lack of movement, to help determine the progression of the rehabilitation plan. Dynamic movement evaluation is always a valuable tool when evaluating horses, and FES allows the observation of this dynamic motion in a controlled environment. In horses that show asymmetrical movement to the FES signal, the goal of further FES treatments is to obtain movement that will become more and more symmetrical, due to the reeducation of the muscle memory through repetition. Most horses that begin FES treatments with an asymmetrical, twisting and rough rotation in the pelvis, showing no clear contraction/relaxation cycle will gradually become more symmetrical with a straight, smooth rotation in the pelvis and a clear contraction/relaxation cycle. The symmetry that develops in the top line can then support a more correct biomechanical loading of the joints in the body as well as in the limbs. Many overuse injuries are due to asymmetrical overloading of the muscles and joints as well as pathological rotation. Therefore, changing the muscle memory to obtain symmetrical movement is a valuable tool in rehabilitation.

Functional electrical stimulation treatment to the neck

FES treatments to the neck can also help reduce spasms and atrophy in the cervical spine region. Six self-adhering electrodes (3 on each side) are placed symmetrically on each side of the neck. Several different arrangements of the electrodes are used based on which muscles of the neck are being addressed. The reaction of the neck muscles to the FES signal is similar to the response of the epaxial and deep muscles of the back. Some horses will have a twist in their neck, as a reaction to the treatment, while other horses will show smooth, straight movement.

Specific sites in the shoulder area and the hindquarters can also be treated unilaterally by placing self-stick electrodes on the targeted site or by holding a pad with electrodes over the site. It is always suggested that if one side of the horse is treated, that the other side is also treated to evaluate and maintain symmetry. Typically, the 'normal' side is treated initially to obtain the parameters of the level of voltage the horse will comfortably accept and the horse's reaction to the treatment, so that a comparison can be made during the treatment of the 'abnormal' side.

Functional electrical stimulation treatment to the limb

For FES treatments on the limbs, a smaller pad is used containing 6 electrodes (3 on each side) that are smaller than those used in the back pad. Upper leg FES treatments of the flexor and extensor muscles of the forearm and gaskin can be used to assist in treating lower-leg tendon and ligament issues. At higher voltages, some horses will flex or extend the lower legs in response to the treatment, however this type of movement is rare. Improvements in the quality of the tendons and ligaments, using ultrasound evaluations, have been limited when the pad is placed on the front or hind upper leg.

FES treatments on the lower legs below the knee and hock will produce more movement in the tendons. The FES signal on the lower legs can be adjusted so that the voltage used will obtain no flexion in the fetlock, a 25% flexion in the fetlock, a 50% flexion in the fetlock, or a complete lifting of the leg in response to the treatment. Using this position of the FES signal on the legs has produced better healing of tendons and ligaments, when evaluated by ultrasound, than on the upper leg. Clinicians using FES on the lower legs have noted an improved rate of healing and a higher quality to the healing tissue. This data is limited and more treatments, with additional data, needs to be collected.

Suspensory ligament, superficial flexor and deep digital flexor strains, sprains and tears have all been treated with FES. The benefits of using FES for these issues includes: an activation of the stretch reflex to assist in fibre alignment during healing, activation of the tissues to reduce oedema, and controlled movement to help reduce excessive fibrin and scar tissue that may develop during healing.

When FES treatments are applied to the limb of the horse, body treatments are performed as well. These body treatments can be to targeted sites such as the shoulders or hindquarters, as well as to the top line. Asymmetries in the body will affect the limb in the same way that asymmetries in the limb will affect the body.

Performance enhancement with functional electrical stimulation

Performance enhancement is another benefit of FES treatment. Horses that are asymmetrical load their body and limbs in a manner that predisposes itself to breakdown. Pathological rotations are the result of incorrect loading, and kinesiological consequences are not far behind these problems. When a practitioner observes an asymmetrical knot of muscle in the loin and this spasm is reduced through the use of FES, the chances of compensatory biomechanical changes in the limbs due to this spasm are reduced. Perhaps this change can then help to reduce a breakdown in the future.

Conclusion

Data from hundreds of case studies, showing thousands of treatments of FES to the top line of the horses have documented improvements pre- and post-FES treatments. These results together with muscle biopsies taken pre- and post-FES treatments and ultrasound measurements of the multifidus taken pre- and post-FES, are all studies being prepared for publication. The positive results from many practitioners throughout the world who are using FES shows that this modality may be worth another look as a tool to assist in moving the science of equine rehabilitation forward.

References

Alon, G., Baker, L., Gersh, M., Kloth, L., Robinson, A.J., Selkowitz, D. and Spielholz N., 2005. Electrotherapeutic terminology in physical therapy: Section on clinical electrophysiology 3rd ed. American Physical Therapy Association, Alexandria, VA, USA, pp. 32-39.

Arnold, P.B., McVey, P.P., Farrell, W.J., Deurloo, T.M. and Grasso, A.R., 1992. Functional electric stimulation: its efficacy and safety in improving pulmonary function and musculoskeletal fitness. Archives of Physical Medicine and Rehabilitation 73: 665-668.

Belda-Lois J.-M., Mena-del Horno S., Bermejo-Bosch I., Moreno, J.C., Pons, J.L., Farins, D., Iosa, M., Molinari, M., Tamburella, F., Ramos, A., Caria, A., Solis-Escalante, T., Brunner, C. and Rea, M., 2011. Rehabilitation of gait after stroke: a review towards a top-down approach. Journal of Neuroengineering and Rehabilitation 8: 66

Carraro, U., Rossini, K., Mayr, W. and Kern, H., 2005. Muscle fiber regeneration in human permanent lower motoneuron denervation: Relevance to safety and effectiveness of FES-training, which induces muscle recovery in SCI subjects. Artificial Organs 29: 187-191.

Faghri, P.D., Yount, J.P., Pesce, W.J., Seetharama, S. and Votto, J.J., 2001. Circulatory hypokinesis and functional electric stimulation during standing in persons with spinal cord injury. Archives of Physical Medicine and Rehabilitation 82: 1587-1595.

Gallien, P., Brissot, R., Eyssette, M., Tell, L., Barat, M., Wiart, L. and Petit, H., 1995. Restoration of gait by functional electrical stimulation for spinal cord injured patients. Paraplegia 33: 660-664.

Granat, M.H., Ferguson, A.C., Andrews, B.J. and Delargy, M., 1993. The role of functional electrical stimulation in the rehabilitation of patients with incomplete spinal cord injury – observed benefits during gait studies. Paraplegia 31: 207-215.

Graupe, D. and Kohn, K.H., 1998. Functional neuromuscular stimulator for short-distance ambulation by certain thoracic-level spinal-cord-injured paraplegics. Surgical Neurology 50: 202-207.

Graupe, D., Cerrel-Bazo, H., Kern, H. and Carraro, U., 2008. Walking performance, medical outcomes and patient training in FES of innervated muscles for ambulation by thoracic-level complete paraplegics. Neurological Research 30: 123-130.

Gregory, C.M. and Bickel, C.S., 2005. Recruitment patterns in human skeletal muscle during electrical stimulation. Physical Therapy 85: 358-364.

Harrelson, G. L., Weber, M.D. and Leaver-Dunn D., 1998. Use of modalities in rehabilitation. In: Andrews, J.R., Harrelson, G.L. and Wilk, K.E. (eds.) Physical rehabilitation of the injured athlete. WB Saunders, Philadelphia, PA, USA, pp. 117-119.

Hines, A., 1994. Functional electrical stimulation for hand opening in spastic hemiplegia. (Electronic Thesis or Dissertation). Available at: https://etd.ohiolink.edu/.

Hyvarinen, A., Tarkka, I.M., Mervaala, E., Paakkonen, A., Valtonen, H. and Nuutinen, J, 2008. Cutaneous electrical stimulation treatment in unresolved facial nerve paralysis: An exploratory study. American Journal of Physical Medicine and Rehabilitation 87: 992-997.

Jacobs, P.L., Johnson, B. and Mahoney, E.T., 2003. Physiologic responses to electrically assisted and frame-supported standing in persons with paraplegia. Journal of Spinal Cord Medicine 26: 384-389.

Johnston, T.E. and Wainwright, S.F., 2011. Cycling with functional electrical stimulation in an adult with spastic diplegic cerebral palsy. Physical Therapy 91: 970-982.

Kawashima, N., Popovic, M.R. and Zivanovic, V., 2008. Effect of intensive functional electrical stimulation therapy on the upper limb motor recovery after stroke: Single case study of a chronic stroke patient. In: Proceedings of the 13th Annual Conference of the International FES Society, Freiburg, Germany, Sept. 21-25, pp. 252-254.

Kern, H., Boncompagni, S., Rossini, K., Mayr, W., Fano, G., Zanin, M.E., Podhorska-Okolow, M., Protasi, F. and Carraro, U., 2004. Long-term denervation in humans causes degeneration of both contractile and excitation-contraction coupling apparatus, which is reversible by functional electrical stimulation (FES): a role for myofiber regeneration? Journal of Neuropathology and Experimental Neurology 63: 919-931.

Kern, H., Hofer, C., Modlin, M., Forstner, C., Raschka-Hogler, D., Mayr, W. and Stohr, H., 2002. Denervated muscles in humans: Limitations and problems of currently used functional electrical stimulation training protocols. Artificial Organs 26: 216-218.

Kern, H., Hofer, C., Modlin, M., Mayr, W., Vindigni, V., Zampieri, S., Boncompagni, S., Protasi, F., and Carraro, U., 2008. Stable muscle atrophy in long-term paraplegics with complete upper motor neuron lesion from 3- to 20-year SCI. Spinal Cord 46: 293-304.

Kern, H., Rossini, K., Carraro, U., Mayr, W., Vogelauer, M., Hoellwarth, U. and Hofer, C., 2005. Muscle biopsies show that FES of denervated muscles reverses human muscle degeneration from permanent spinal motoneuron lesion. Journal of Rehabilitation Research and Development 42: 43-53.

Krause, P., Szecsi, J. and Straube, A., 2007. FES cycling reduces spastic muscle tone in a patient with multiple sclerosis. Neurorehabilitation 22: 335-337.

Lim, J.Y. and Han, T.R., 2010. Effect of electromyostimulation on apoptosis-related factors in denervation and reinnervation of rat skeletal muscles. Muscle and Nerve 42: 422-430.

Marqueste, T., Decherchi, P., Desplanches, D., Favier, R., Grelot, L. and Jammes, Y., 2006. Chronic electrostimulation after nerve repair by self-anastomosis: Effects on the size, the mechanical, histochemical and biochemical muscle properties. Acta Neuropathologica 111: 589-600.

Masani, K. and Popovic, M.R., 2011. The basis of electrical stimulation: Functional electrical stimulation in rehabilitation and neurorehabilitation In: Kramme, R., Hoffmann, K.-P. and Pozos, R. (eds.) Springer handbook of medical technology. Springer-Verlag, Berlin, Germany, pp. 877-896.

Mirbagheri, M.M., Ladouceur, M., Barbeau, H. and Kearney, R.E., 2002. The effects of long-term FES-assisted walking on intrinsic and reflex dynamic stiffness in spastic spinal-cord-injured subjects. IEEE Transactions on Neural Systems Rehabilitation Engineering 10: 280-289.

Mushahwar, V.K., Jacobs, P.L., Normann, R.A., Triolo, R.J. and Kleitman, N., 2007. New functional electrical stimulation approaches to standing and walking. Journal of Neural Engineering 4: S181-197.

Pollack, S.F., Axen, K., Spielholz, N., Levin, N., Haas, F. and Ragnarsson, K.T., 1989. Aerobic training effects of electrically induced lower extremity exercises in spinal cord injured people. Archives of Physical Medicine and Rehabilitation 70: 214-219.

Popovic, D.B., Sinkjær and T., Popovic, M.B., 2009. Electrical stimulation as a means for achieving recovery of function in stroke patients. NeuroRehabilitation 25: 45-58.

Rattay F., Resatz S., Lutter P., Minassian K., Jilge B. and Dimitrijevic M.R., 2003. Mechanisms of electrical stimulations with neural prosethesis. Neuromodulation 6: 42-56.

Schils, S.J., 2009. Review of electrotherapy devices for use in veterinary medicine. In: Proceedings of the 55th Annual Convention of the American Association of Equine Practitioners, Las Vegas, NV, USA, Dec. 5-9, pp. 68-73.

Schils, S.J., 2010. Functional electrical stimulation (FES) for use in equine medicine. In: Lindner, A. (ed.) Performance diagnosis and purchase examination of elite sport horses. Wageningen Academic Publishers, Wageningen, the Netherlands, pp. 103-108.

Schils, S.J., 2012. Functional electrical stimulation for muscle wasting in equine rehabilitation. In: Proceedings of the 7th International Symposium on Veterinary Rehabilitation and Physical Therapy, Vienna, Austria, August 15-18, p. 97.

Stackhouse, S., 2008. Electrical stimulation of muscle of control of movement and posture. In: Robinson, A.J. and Snyder-Mackler, L. (eds.) Clinical electrophysiology: electrotherapy and electrophysiologic testing. Lippincott Williams and Wilkins, Baltimore, MD, USA, pp. 239-262.

Stefanovska, A., Vodovnik, L., Gros, N., Rebersek, S. and Acimovic-Janezic, R., 1989. FES and spasticity. IEEE Transactions on Biomedical Engineering 36: 738-745.

Szecsi, J. and Schiller, M., 2009. FES-propelled cycling of SCI subjects with highly spastic leg musculature. Neurorehabilitation 24: 243-253.

Thrasher, T.A., Zivanovic, V., McIlroy, W. and Popovic, M.R., 2008. Rehabilitation of reaching and grasping function in severe hemiplegic patients using functional electrical stimulation therapy. Neurorehabilitation and Neural Repair 22: 706-714.

Wang, R.Y., Yang, Y.R., Tsai, M.W., Wang, W.T.J. and Chan, R.C., 2002. Effects of functional electric stimulation on upper limb motor function and shoulder range of motion in hemiplegic patients. American Journal of Physical Medicine and Rehabilitation 81: 283-290.

Yarkony, G.M., Jaeger, R.J., Roth, E., Kralj, A.R. and Quintern, J., 1990. Functional neuromuscular stimulation for standing after spinal cord injury. Archives of Physical Medicine and Rehabilitation 71: 201-206.

Can fascia improve the performance and general health condition in horses?

Vibeke S. Elbrønd[1] *and Rikke M. Schultz*[2]
University of Copenhagen, Faculty of Veterinary Science, Department of Veterinary Clinical and Animal Sciences, Section of Anatomy and Biochemistry, Grønnegårdsvej 7, 1870 Frederiksberg C, Denmark; [2]*RMS Equine practice, Karlebovej 22, 2980 Kokkedal, Denmark; vse@sund.ku.dk*

Introduction

Training, treatment and rehabilitation of the locomotion system in horses has for many years focused mainly on muscles, skeleton and joints. Only minor attention has been paid to fascia (connective tissue), and it can be speculated why. Fascial structures such as tendons, ligaments and joint capsules has had the highest priority, and it is well known that rehabilitation of these structures span over many months up to years if ever fully recovered and restituted. There has been a lack of research in other fascia structures. Perhaps due to the perception that the structures are constructed of a more or less inert material with only a mechanical function in relation to the locomotion system. In the veterinary world surgeons cut it, repose it and suture it. Traumatized skin, muscles or other structures heal by exchanging damaged tissue with stiff and hard connective tissue forming a scar, which is accepted to be the final state of a healing process.

In the last decade interest towards the fascia has increased exponentially and many exciting and fascinating results have improved our understanding and knowledge of how vital fascia interactions with the central nervous system as well as other structures are (e.g. in the locomotion system), and how lively and plastic the connective tissue can be in many ways. Some researchers even name it the 'Cinderella'-tissue due to the continuously increasing number of fascinating results which turn up and present the numerous transformations it can undergo – showing a new pretty face day for day (Schleip *et al.*, 2012).

What is the common knowledge about fascia

Veterinary anatomy is as well as human anatomy very modest when presenting the fasciae and regard them only as macroscopically and visible anatomical structures. In most textbooks fasciae are defined as sheets of connective tissue made out of dense and irregularly woven collagenous fibres and equipped with a physical characteristic as high tensile and multidirectional strong tissue. The fasciae enwrap the body, the muscles and their supportive structures. Two major fasciae are described: (1) a superficial sheet right underneath the skin – like a full body swim-suit; and (2) a more profound sheet closely attached to the surface of the muscles forming fingerlike projections between and into the muscles. This 'common knowledge' of a rather inert but strong tissue has been evident for many years. Not that the knowledge of other types of connective tissues and the presence of neuroreceptors within the tissue has been forgotten, but the awareness and understanding of how important and essential the interactions within the tissue itself and with other structures has just taken its start and much more is to come.

It will be relevant in this paper to question if veterinarians, riders and therapists can have any advantage of the present knowledge about fascia. The horse has not been the first choice as lab animal for research studies, but the situation is changing and studies are on their way. The intension of this article is to bring forward some new knowledge and to evaluate the role of the fascia (connective tissue) in the horse.

Basic knowledge: old and new

To better understand todays´ perception of the fascia some basic but important concepts are presented. First of all the terminology has been changed. Now the name 'fascia' includes all types of soft connective tissue.

Connective tissue

Connective tissue has its origin from the mesoderm, and already at a very early embryonic stage (day 17) the mesoderm divides into an intra- and extra-embryonic portion (Hyttel *et al.* 2010). The extra embryonic mesoderm splits into a splanchnic and somatic layer, which respectively develop into the serosal layer around the viscera and at the walls of the body cavities. The other portion, the intra embryonic mesoderm now mentioned as the paraxial mesoderm, develops into a variety of cell types such as blood stem cells, myoblasts, fibrocytes, chondrocytes, osteocytes, mast cells, fat cells, endothelial cells and reticular cells. When joining together the cells form many different tissues such as fat tissue, loose interstitial tissue (subcutaneous, subpleural, subperitoneal tissue), strong and tight connective tissue (fasciae, ligaments, tendons, aponeuroses, joint capsules, retinaculae), cartilage and bone. All these tissues have a cellular and an extracellular (matrix) portion. In the matrix portion the fibres (elastic, collagen and reticular) are arranged in conjunction with interfibrillar proteins (glucosaminoglycans and proteoglycans) and water. The proportion of fibres, proteins and water defines the physical appearance of the tissue, e.g. loose connective tissue, dense connective tissue, cartilage or bone. In the cellular portion mature as well as immature cells are present. The immature cells are the 'active' ones. They are able to renew and replace damaged and worn out collagen fibres, but at a limited speed. Magnusson *et al.* (2010) measured that after exercise fibroblasts in tendons needed at least 36-48 hours to replace the amount of damaged and worn out collagen fibres.

Connective tissue is distributed everywhere in the body (Figure 1), and if all types of 'organ cells' (e.g. muscle-, bone-, liver-, kidney-cells) are removed a three dimensional and very delicate but complicated network of connective tissue remains in a full body shape. With respect to the locomotion system, Myers (2009) describes the body like a big sac with 600 muscle compartments. It is now possible to follow the fibres in the network from one end of the body to the other – from toe to head. Other structures of the locomotion system (muscles, tendons, bones, etc.) are to be thought about as being 'inserted' into this network as described by Myers (2009). If we now focus e.g. on a muscle the fascial relation is found even at the cellular level as illustrated in Figure 1. Connective tissue enwraps every single muscle cell and is named the endomysium (Figure 1, d). The endomysium from several cells fuses into the perimysium (Figure 1, f), visible as thin white lines in the adult muscle, and outermost upon the muscle body is the epimysium (Figure 1, b). In one end the epimysium transforms into a muscle origo (Figure 1, g), and in the other end to an insertion (a tendon, Figure 1, c). Both ends fuse with the periosteum on the surface of the bones (Figure 1d).

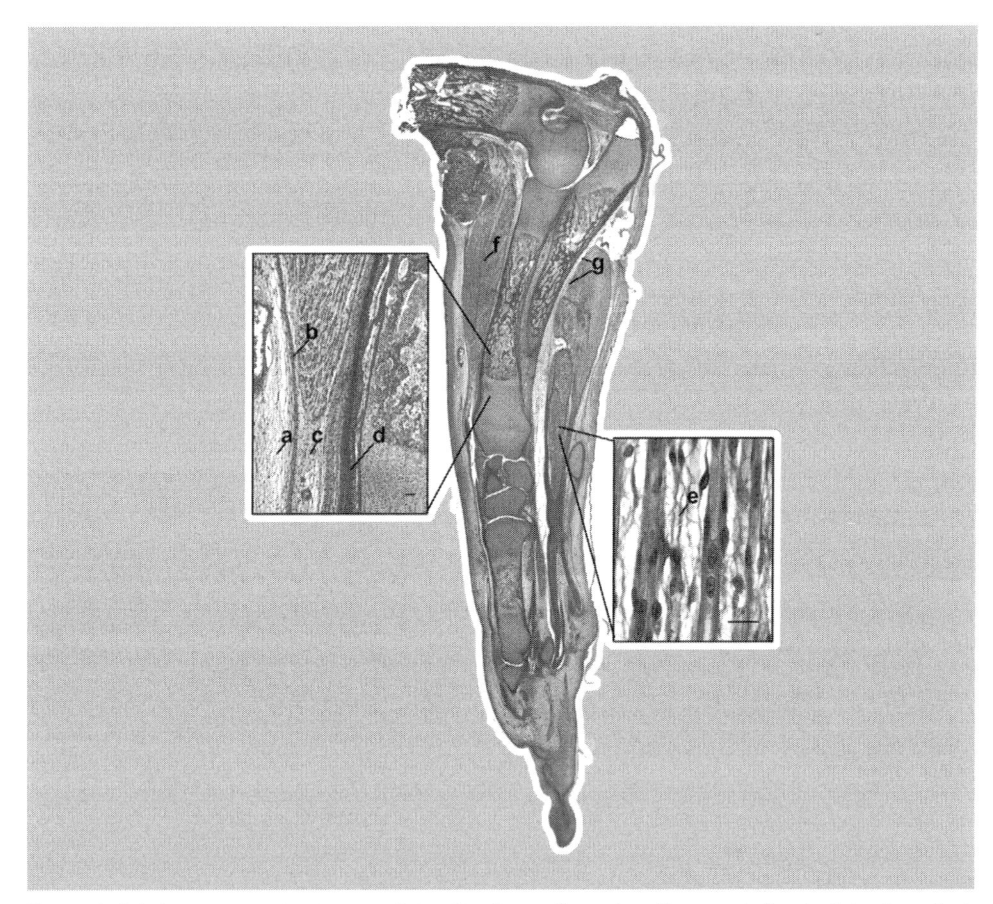

Figure 1. A light microscopic picture of the distal part from the elbow and distal of the front limb from a pig embryo (7 weeks old). Preformed bones, joints, muscles, tendons and ligaments are seen. In the insert to the left the primitive connective tissue is present in the already preformed structures. Notice how the different layers are merged more or less unlimited into each other. The darker stained areas represent zones in which the amount of collageneous fibres are so high that they are visible after staining. In the right insert (high magnification of skeletal muscle) the connective tissue is localized in between the muscle fibres (endomysium). (a) profound fascia, (b) perimysium, (c) tendon tissue from the extensor muscle, (d) periost, (e) endomysium, (f) epimysial sheet in the extensor muscle. Magnification bar in the inserts represent 10 μm.

Tensegrity

Tensegrity, which has been introduced by the designer Buckminster Fuller (1975), is another concept to be presented. The word is a composition of 'tension and integrity'. It describes how a structure can hold its form when balanced 'tension' and 'compression' forces are combined. This phenomenon can be visualized with a model as seen in Figure 2a. It is constructed of pins arranged in a three dimensional lattice with rubber bands in between. The compression elements (pins) do not touch each other and are kept in place by the tension elements (rubber bands). If pressed into, the structure loses its original shape and the force is distributed to the other elements as seen in Figure 2b. When we transfer the model to the locomotion system, in which the bones are the compression elements and the connective tissue the rubber bands, it is now easier to understand, why injury or hypertension in one end of the body can cause symptoms in the other.

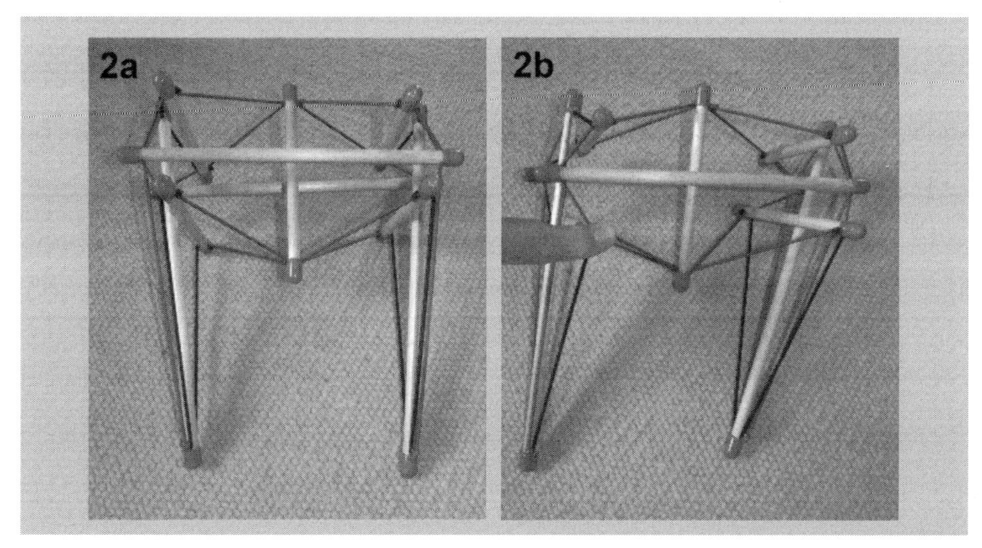

Figure 2. (a) A tensegrity model with compression elements (pins) and tension elements (rubber bands) attaching the end of the pins. In conjunction they create a system of forces in balance, which keep up the shape of the model. (b) Forces from outside (finger pressure) interrupt the balance, the internal forces are redistributed and the shape of the model has changed.

Sensation in the fascia

Fascia is found to be one of the best developed sensory organs in the body. Compared to muscles the fascial network possesses a ten times higher quantity of sensory nerve receptors (Van der Wal, 2009). Four major types of receptors are present in the fasciae. Three of them are myelinated receptors: Golgi, Pacini and Ruffini bodies. They are found to be related to the proprioception (Stecco *et al.*, 2007) and inform the brain about stretch, shear, pressure, position and balance in the body. They are the receptors addressed in manual therapies and skin taping. The fourth receptor type is the unmyelinated interoceptive free nerve ending (slow C-fibre). The fibre is present in an innumerable amount in the fascia particularly in the periosteum, endo- and perimysium and the visceral connective tissue. They are the most important source for interoception, the sense where the brain is informed about the physiological condition in the tissue (e.g. pH, oxygen, blood flow). Impulses from proprioception and interoception are both transported to the brain but treated in two different locations respectively the somatocortex and the insula (Craig, 2009). The somatocortex treats the proprioceptive informations and responds to actions and movements in the locomotion system. The insula region is related to the homeostatic needs in the body and the sensations are very often associated with behavioural motivations that are essential to maintaining the body needs (Berlucchi and Aglioti 2010). Bertolucci (2011) suggested that pandiculation (stretching of the fasciae in the body) and yawning observed in both animals and humans could be a neurologic reset of fascia when the body is transferred from one physiological condition to another, e.g. asleep – awake.

Myofascial chains

In the locomotion system tight connections and relations between fasciae, muscles and bony/skeletal structures give rise to shorter 'local' and longer 'full body' chains with functional interactions named: myofascial kinetic chains. The myofascial chains are arranged in well-defined and specific lines in the body and attach to bony/skeletal structures like the tensegrity system mentioned earlier. The system is fine-tuned, it balances the body and influences the body posture not only in standing position but also in motion, therefore the name kinetic trains. If a line is disrupted (e.g. by a trauma or a dysfunction) the balance and distribution of the internal forces are changed and thereby also the shape and posture of the body. This is a condition which is very often observed by riders, trainers, therapists and veterinarians and can be difficult to sort out and understand. At this point knowledge about the myofascial lines might help to understand the functional relationship in the body and to clear up the source of problem.

In the book 'Anatomy trains' Thomas Myers (2009) presented ten myofascial kinetic trains, which were dissected and isolated in the human body. The trains consisted of functionally related myofascial structures (fasciae, ligaments, aponeuroses, muscles and periost). Several of them had a span from one end of the body to the other. Specific for the trains were that (1) all fibres in a train had the same functional direction; (2) the fibres and structures were located in the same level of the body; and (3) the structures in the train had a 'similar/synergistic function'. Myers (2009) also presented how imbalances/disturbances within and between the trains influenced the posture of the human body. Of the ten human trains three were found to be superficial and reached from head to toe, four were related to the arms, one went profound through the inner thoracic and abdominal cavity and two trains were helical and crossed over between the left and the right side of the body. The chains were also found to interact. This interaction is one of thc keypoints in order to understand how forces are distributed, when balance is broken.

At the Veterinary Faculty, University of Copenhagen, R.M. Schultz, and undersigned have dissected and studied more than 20 horses of different age and breed and verified eight myofascial kinetic chains (unpublished data). With some exceptions the horse lines mirrored the human trains, and the differences we found might very well be explained by the species differences. We did some renaming to the concept. The word 'trains' was changed to 'chains' in order to underline the tight collaboration between the structures throughout the body. Additionally some of the chains were renamed in order to meet the veterinary nomenclature which is used due to the difference in posture between the quadruped horse and the biped human.

Superficial lines

Three superficial chains (from head to heel) were identified and verified in the horses. The superficial dorsal line (SDL), the superficial ventral line (SVL) and the lateral line (LL) (Figure 3a). The SDL comprised structures involved in extension of head, neck, back, hip, and hock and flexion of the knee and foot/tarsus. The SVL comprised structures which flex the head, neck, back, hip and hock and extend the knee and foot, and the LL structures were involved in lateral bending/flexion of the head, neck back, lumbar area and hip and abduction of the hind leg.

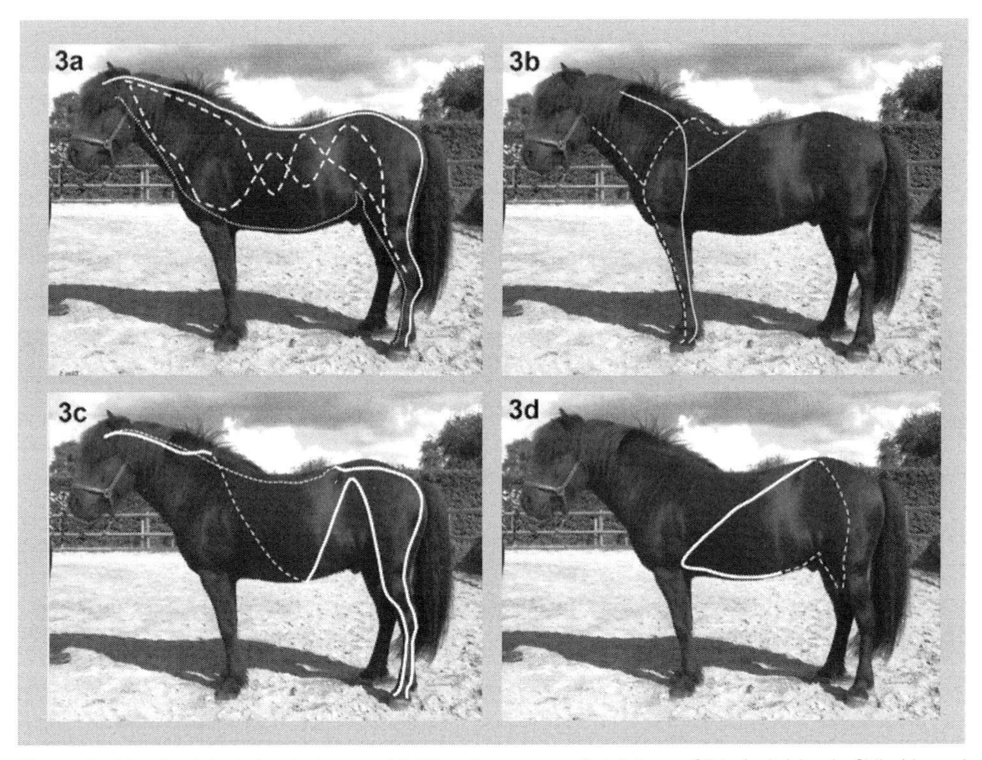

Figure 3. Myofascial chains in horse. (a) The three superficial lines: SDL (solid line), SVL (dotted line) and LL (dashed line). (b) The two front limb lines: FLRL (solid line) and FLPL (dashed line). (c, d) The helical lines: spiral line (SL) and functional line (FL), respectively. The solid part of the lines is located on the visible side of the horse and the dashed line on the opposite side.

Functionally the SDL and SVL act as antagonists around the horizontal axis of the horse (body flexion and extension). Very importantly the lines connect in the head and the toe of the hind leg. Biomechanically the interaction between these two lines is very similar to the 'bow-string' concept (Slijper, 1946) in which the dorsal (top) and the ventral (bottom) line balance each other in order to stabilize the flexibility of the trunk. In contrast to the bow-string-theory, the myofascial chains (SDL and SVL) interact in the full body length from the head and neck to the distal part of the hind leg. This improves the model as the structures in addition are all well known to impose high forces and influence on the balance of the body.

The LL works around the vertical body axis and collaborates with both the SDL and the SVL from head to toe. This feature is expressed by the more or less diploid appearance of the LL, in which the upper part (dorsal) collaborates with the SDL and the lower (ventral) with the SVL. The three lines in conjunction outline and support the body in a closely integrated three dimensional and balanced system in standing and in motion.

Front limb lines

In the front limbs we dissected and isolated two major lines: A front limb protraction line (FLRL) and a front limb retraction line (FLPL) (Figure 3b). The lines describe the movements of the front limb, protraction and retraction, and include also the movements of the scapula, parts of the upper trunk and lower neck. The two lines act as antagonists and balance the movement and posture of the front limb. In balance they keep the front limbs in a vertical position under the standing body. If, e.g. the retraction line is tensed up (as often seen in horses with biomechanical problems in the trunk and hindquarter), the front limbs are forced under the body. A high stress is then applied to the vital structures in the distal part of the foot such as superficial and deep flexor tendons; check (accessory) ligaments; proximal and distal sesamoid bones and ligaments. Very important to mention here is that the front limb lines in motion interact with several of the other lines.

Helical lines

The two helical lines, spiral line (SL) and functional line (FL) (Figure 3c) have one or more crossings of the midline. They hereby connect the right and left half of the body. The lines establish movements around the sagittal body axis, the axial rotation. The two lines are very active in cross coordination as seen in trot, three beat gallop, toelt in Icelandic Horses or 4-beat gaits in gaited horses etc. In motion the helical lines were found to be in very close relation with the front limb lines, and the question is if they in these situations are to be regarded as an extension of the helical lines.

Profound line

The deep ventral line is the eighth line and in our opinion possibly the most potent of the lines as it comprises the fascia lining the inside of the thoracic and abdominal cavity (Figure 3d). The deep ventral line connects 'inside with outside' at the thoracic and pelvic apertures. Several of the muscles and structures located within the cavities (e.g. m. psoas major, psoas minor, m. longus colli) are involved in stabilization of the spine and neck. Disturbances in the DVL might turn out into posture problems.

Perspectives

With the improved understanding of fasciae in general and the myofascial kinetic lines as fascia layers, which can tighten up and disrupt the body balance, it becomes more and more clear that it is necessary to be able to treat the connective tissue. This is to be done in order to reestablish body balance and homeostasis in the fasia tissue and to optimize the biomechanics in the horses. In this context it is also important to understand how and when the fascia tissue can change and how much the changes affect the locomotion system. It is a difficult task to evaluate due to the rich innervation of the fascia system and to the large individual variations in the perception between horses. Most important is to prevent. To be aware of the sources of damage and not to neglect the possible negative effect of scars in the skin and muscle, soft tissue trauma and to observe and evaluate the body posture and treat before 'things settle'.

Acknowledgments

The studies of the myofascial chains have been financially supported by 'The International Veterinary Chiropractic Association' (IVCA) and 'The Foundation for Promotion of Veterinary Science'.

References

Berlucchi, G. and Aglioti, S.M., 2010. The body in the brain revisited. Experimental Brain Research 200: 25-35.

Bertolucci L.F., 2011. Pandiculation: nature's way of maintaining the functional integrity of the myofascial system? Journal of Bodywork and Movement Therapies 15: 268-280.

Craig, A. D., 2009. How do you fell now? The anterior insula and human awareness. Nature Reviews Neuroscience 10: 59-70.

Fuller, B., 1975. Synergetic. Macmillan, New York, NY, USA.

Hyttel, P., Sinowatz, F. and Vejlsted, M., 2010. Essentials of domestic animal embryology. Saunders Elsevier, New York, NY, USA, pp. 79-94.

König, H.E. and Liebich, H-G., 2004. Veterinary Anatomy of Domestic Mammals. 4th ed. Schattauer GmbH, Stuttgart, Germany.

Magnusson, S.P., Langberg, H. and Kjaer, M., 2010. The pathogenesis of tendinopathy: balancing the response to loading. Nature Reviews Rheumatology 6: 262-268

Myers, T., 2009. Anatomy trains. Myofascial meridians for manual and movement therapists. 2nd ed. Churchill Livingstone, Elsevier Health Sciences, Philadelphia, PA, USA.

Schleip, R., Findley, T.W., Chaitow, L. and Huijing P.A., 2012. Fascia: the tensional network of the human body. The Science and Clinical Applications in manual movement therapy. 1st ed. Elsevier Health Science, Edinburg, UK.

Sleijper, E.J., 1946. Comparative biologic-anatomical investigations on the vertebral column and spinal musculature of mammals. NV. Noord-Hollandsche Uitgevers Maatschapp IJ, Amsterdam, the Netherlands.

Stecco, C., Gagey, O. and Belloni, A., 2007. Anatomy of the deep fascia of the upper limb. Second part: study of innervation. Morphologie 91: 38-43.

Van der Wal, J.C., 2009. The architecture of the connective tissue in the musculoskeletal system: an often overlooked functional parameter as to proprioception in the locomotor apparatus. Int J Ther Massage Bodywork 2(4): 9-23.

Expanded abstracts

Evaluation of post-exercise recovery in eventing horses

J.F. Azevedo, A.C.T. Miranda, M.T. Ramos, C.A.A. Oliveira, F.G.F. Padilha, V.P. Silva, C.D. Baldani and F.Q. Almeida
Veterinary Institute. Universidade Federal Rural do Rio de Janeiro, BR 465, Km 07. Seropédica, RJ 23897-97, Brazil; falmeida@ufrrj.br

Take home message

An exponential regression equation describes the reduction of plasma lactate concentration after incremental speed tests at field or treadmill best, while the haematocrit reduction was best described by a linear regression equation. The measured plasma activities of aspartate aminotransferase (AST) creatine kinase (CK) allow to conclude that the incremental speed tests used did not cause muscle injury in horses.

Introduction

Most studies about exercise physiology are performed on a treadmill due to the readiness and standardization of conditions as well as easy access to the horses during and after exercise (Martin *et al.*, 2004). The field tests are carried out in exercise conditions similar to those observed during training and competitions (Van Erck *et al.*, 2007). The most used variables to determinate the workload during the performance evaluation tests in horses are heart rate, plasma lactate and oxygen consumption. The present study aimed to obtain modelling data of plasma lactate and glucose concentrations and haematocrit in eventing horses after incremental speed tests on the field and on a high speed treadmill.

Material and methods

The study was carried out at the Horse's Performance Evaluation Laboratory at the Brazilian Army Cavalry School. The tests were performed with a high speed treadmill in an acclimatized room and the field tests were performed on a grass track. Eight eventing Brazilian

Sport Horses were used, five males and three females, with mean age of 7.4 ± 1.2 years old, and average body weight of 478.6 ± 34.1 kg.

The protocol for the incremental speed test on the treadmill was adapted from Hodgson and Rose (1994), and consisted of 10 minutes of warm up, at walk and trot; followed, with the treadmill inclined at 4%, by gallops, starting at a 5.0 m/s speed, increasing the speed in 1.0 m/s every minute until 10.0 m/s (5.0, 6.0, 7.0, 8.0, 9.0 and 10.0 m/s). At the end of the test, the recovery was proceeded with 4 minutes of trot (4.0 m/s) and 6 minutes of walk (1.7 m/s), without inclination of the treadmill. The protocol used on the field test was adapted from the model proposed by Wilson *et al.* (1983), and consisted of 10 minutes of warm up, at walk and trot, followed by 4 steps of one minute at 5.0, 7.0, 8.0 and 10.0 m/s, with 3 minute intervals of walk for the horse's recovery between each step.

In all tests, basal blood samples were obtained previously to the first meal, from the left jugular vein with tubes containing EDTA or sodium fluoride for analysis of haematocrit, lactate and glucose, respectively. To evaluate the recovery of the tests, blood samples were obtained 10, 20 and 30 minutes after the end of the last step. In order to evaluate the muscular damage caused by the tests, blood samples were collected from left jugular vein at the end of each step and 1, 2, 6, 12 and 24 hours after, in an anticoagulant free tube for analysis of AST and CK. The haematocrit was performed in an automatic cell counter. Lactate, glucose, AST and CK analysis were performed in a spectrophotometer.

Values of plasma lactate, haematocrit and glucose concentrations were adjusted by regression analysis to evaluate the effect of the treatment as a function of time after tests. The variables CK and AST were tested for homoscedasticity and homogeneity by Cochran and Bartlett´s test and for normality by Lilliefors test. Only the variable CK did not assume normal distribution and, therefore, was transformed to logarithm base 10. AST and CK values were subjected to analysis of variance as a split-splot and the means compared by Tukey test at 5% probability, with the Statistics Analysis and Planning of Research Software (SISVAR).

Results

The values of plasma lactate, haematocrit and glucose before and after the tests indicated a reduction to basal values 60 minutes after exercises, while plasma glucose concentration increased after tests (Table 1).

The best fit model of plasma lactate concentration at recovery from the treadmill and the field tests was described by an exponential equation. The incremental speed field test presented a determination coefficient of 0.58, which was lower than the coefficient of the incremental speed treadmill test of 0.73, indicating greater consistency between the results of horses when tests were conducted on high speed treadmill (Table 2). Marlin *et al.* (1991) evaluated the removal of lactate after seven speed tests and observed linear decrease response of lactate concentration, and that the reduction rate of lactate concentration did not vary with speed.

Regarding the haematocrit, differences among the coefficients of determination of linear and exponential functions were of little importance. Thus, the regression equation that best described the relationship between the haematocrit and the time of recovery after progressive test was linear which is the simplest model (Table 3).

Table 1. Plasma lactate and glucose concentrations, and haematocrit (means ± standard deviation) in horses after tests.

	During test		**After test**		
Tests	**Basal**	**Last step**	**10 min**	**30 min**	**60 min**
Plasma lactate (mmol/l)					
Field	0.5±0.2	3.8±0.7	6.1±1.2	1.6±0.8	0.9±0.4
Treadmill	0.5±0.1	6.9±2.1	9.1±2.9	4.8±2.3	2.6±1.3
Haematocrit (%)					
Field	34.6±3.5	52.0±5.3	41.0±5.0	37.9±5.7	34.6±3.4
Treadmill	34.8±3.2	59.1±4.1	51.4±5.9	44.7±3.9	38.1±2.9
Glucose (mmol/l)					
Field	5.28±0.34	5.61±0.46	5.94±0.32	6.67±0.44	7.22±0.71
Treadmill	5.44±0.42	6.22±1.44	6.11±0.91	7.34±1.43	6.94±0.88

Table 2. Regression equation and determination coefficient (r^2) for the relationship between plasma lactate and time after exercise tests.

Exercise test	Relation	Equation	r^2
Field	Linear	y=4.09-0.070x	0.46
	Exponential	$y=0.5067e^{-0.0134x}$	0.58
Treadmill	Linear	y=7.25-0.117x	0.56
	Exponential	$y=0.8629e^{-0.0159x}$	0.73

Table 3. Regression equation and determination coefficient (r^2) for the relationship between hematocrit and time after exercise tests.

Exercise test	Relation	Equation	r^2
Field	Linear	y=47.73-0.25x	0.47
	Exponential	$y=0.1674e^{-0.0026x}$	0.49
Treadmill	Linear	y=56.70-0.34x	0.75
	Exponential	$y=1.7545e^{-0.0032x}$	0.79

There was no difference ($P>0.05$) among mean values of plasma glucose concentration during recovery time, so it was not possible to adjust plasma glucose during recovery from exercise test with a regression equation. Mean plasma glucose concentration during recovery of incremental speed tests in the field or on the treadmill was 6.61 mmol/l.

There was no significant difference ($P>0.05$) in AST between tests, and no interaction effects between time and tests. There were differences ($P<0.05$) in AST among the times of the post-test (Table 4), with an increase 2 hours after exercise peaking at 6 hours after the end of the test, with an average of 379 U/l. All values are within the reference values ranging from 100 to 400 U/L (Rose and Hodgson, 1994).

There were significant differences ($P>0.05$) in CK among times, and the highest concentration of CK was observed 6 hours after the test, with an average of 418.93 U/L (Table 4). Two hours after tests, CK begins to increase exceeding the reference values of 100 to 300 U/L

Table 4. Aspartate aminotransferase (AST) and creatine kinase (CK) (means ± standard deviation) after exercise tests.

	Last step	1h	2h	6h	12h	24h
AST (U/l)	347±47[c]	340±58[c]	351±54[b]	379±61[a]	355±51[b]	332±49[c]
CK (U/l)	235±31[a]	288±50[b]	322±66[b]	419±49[c]	303±45[b]	249±53[a]

Means on lines followed by the same lower case letters do not differ by Tukey test ($P>0.05$).

(Rose and Hodgson, 1994). No difference was observed in the AST and CK concentrations indicating that no muscle injuries occurred in both tests.

Conclusions

After incremental speed tests in the field and on treadmill an exponential regression equation described the reduction of plasma lactate concentration best, while the reduction of haematocrit was better described by a linear regression equation. The measured activities of AST and CK allow to conclude that the incremental speed tests used did not cause muscle injury in horses.

References

Marlin, D.J., Harris, R.C. and Snow, D.H., 1991. Rates of blood lactate disappearance following exercise of different intensities. In: Persson, S.G.B., Lindholm, A. and Jeffcott, L.B. (eds.) Equine Exercise Physiology, 3rd ed., ICEEP Publications, Davis, CA, USA, pp. 188-195.

Martin, B.B., Davidson, E.J., Durando, D.D. and Birks, D.D., 2004. In: Hinchcliff, K.W., Kaneps, A.J. and Geor, R.J. (eds.) Equine sport medicine and surgery: basic and clinical sciences of the equine athlete. Saunders Company, Philadelphia, PA, USA, pp. 27-44.

Rose, R.J. and Hodgson, D.R., 1994. Hematology and Biochemistry. In: Hodgson, D.R. and Rose, R.J. (ed.) The athletic horse: Principles and practice of equine sports medicine, W.B. Saunders, Philadelphia, PA, USA, pp. 63-78.

Van Erck, E., Votion, D.M., Serteyn, D. and Art, T., 2007. Evaluation of oxygen consumption during field exercise tests in Standardbred trotters. Equine and Comparative Exercise Physiology 4: 43-49.

Wilson, R.G., Isler, R.B. and Thornton, J.R., 1983. Heart rate, lactic acid production and speed during a standardised exercise test in Standardbred horses. In: Snow, D.H., Persson, S.G.B. and Rose, J.R. (eds.) Equine Exercise Physiology. Burlington Press, Cambridge, UK, pp. 487-496.

Assessment of a novel antioxidant supplement enriched with fish oils on the muscle cell physiology of exercising Thoroughbred horses

M. Dowling[1], A.D. Fahey[2], V.P. Gath[1], C.A. Williams[3], V. Duggan[1] and F.J. Mulligan[1]
[1]School of Veterinary Medicine, University College Dublin, Belfield, Dublin 4, Ireland; [2]School of Agriculture and Food Science, University College Dublin, Belfield, Dublin 4, Ireland; [3]Rutgers, the State University, Department of Animal Science, Bartlet Hall, 84 Lipman Drive, New Brunswick, NJ 08901-8525, USA; maureen.dowling@ucdconnect.ie

Take home message

This study involved the use of a supplement containing a mixture of natural plant derived material with antioxidant properties, protected vitamin C and chelated selenium, enriched with encapsulated fish oils. Decreased glutathione peroxidase (GSH-Px) levels in the control group at the end of the blood sampling period following exercise in week 7 of supplementation and lower creatine kinase (CK) levels in the treatment group throughout the training programme seem to indicate a beneficial effect of a supplementation with natural exogenous ingredients.

Introduction

Oxidation is a normal metabolic process which allows organisms to convert nutrients into energy for everyday function and performance. Oxidation however, produces free radicals and reactive oxygen species (ROS), which can be detrimental to cells if produced in high enough amounts. The cell membranes of skeletal muscle cells are particularly sensitive to damage by ROS. Normally antioxidants competently prevent free radical damage by preventing their excessive formation, by inactivating them and by aiding the repair of damaged tissue. Oxidative stress is a disturbance of the equilibrium between antioxidants and oxidants, in favour of oxidants. It occurs when the antioxidant system is overwhelmed by an increased oxidant burden of ROS or by a reduced antioxidant supply. This imbalance is common in horses during exercise, at the beginning of training programmes and especially during recovery from exercise (Avellini *et al.*, 1999). Supplementation with antioxidants is vital to rebalance this equilibrium (Urso and Clarkson, 2003). Reducing the extent of muscle damage caused by these free radicals and reducing the recovery time after an exercise event could yield advantages to owners, trainers and the horse. The aim of this experiment was to test the efficacy of a novel supplement for conferring improved antioxidant status and muscle cell physiology on Thoroughbred horses in pre-training stages.

Materials and methods

A cross-over experimental design was used; encompassing ten individually housed, unfit Thoroughbred mares (5.6 ± 1.05 years). Two diets were fed: (1) the treatment diet (TRT); containing a mixture of natural plant derived material with antioxidant properties, vitamin C, chelated selenium (Se) and starch encapsulated fish oils; and (2) the control diet (CON); a commercially available equine feed including the most commonly used antioxidants in equine feed (α-tocopherol 300 IU/kg and Se 0.75 mg/kg). The diets were designed to provide 50% of the energy required from hay (perennial ryegrass) and 50% from concentrates with an average intake of 4.41 ± 0.35 kg/day of concentrates and 5.38 kg/day of hay. Feeding rates were determined by assessing the energy requirements of horses at a moderate training level of work for appropriate body weights (NRC, 2007). The mares were exercised and fed the diets for two periods of eight weeks. A wash out period of 16 weeks was used between experimental periods, to allow fitness levels to return to pre-trial basal levels and for the animals to attain a similar antioxidant status to that with which they commenced the study.

Prior to beginning each experimental phase, all horses were tested for their inherent fitness levels. Each horse underwent identical exercise treadmill tests and maximum heart-rate (HR_{max}) values were recorded as previously described by Williams and Carlucci (2006). The time to reach HR_{max} was used to block animals on inherent fitness before being randomly assigned to treatments within the blocks.

The experimental training programme was such that horses worked to 60-70% of maximum heart rate on a ten-horse capacity exerciser, every day for the eight weeks. Heart rates were monitored using Polar Equine Equipment.

Daily exercise regimes began and finished each day with 15 minutes of warm up and cool down at 2.2 m/s. Exercise stage durations ranged from 20 minutes in week 4 (3 m/s) up to 40 minutes in week 8 (4.5 m/s). However, the duration of exercise was increased once per week on sample day by 30% in week 4, 35% in week 5, 40% in week 6, 45% in week 7 and by 50% in week 8 to increase exercise induced oxidative stress in the horses.

Blood sampling was carried out in the middle of each week from weeks 4-8 of the periods, however only samples from week 4, 7 and 8 were analysed. Samples were harvested via jugular venipunture and taken pre-exercise (PRE), immediately post-exercise (POST), 30 minutes post-exercise (30MIN), 3 hours post-exercise (3HR) and 24 hours post-exercise (24HR). Samples were analysed fresh or immediately centrifuged for 10 minutes at 1,500 × *g* at 4 °C and stored at -80 °C. Erythrocyte lysate was prepared and aliquoted as described by (Lamprecht and Williams, 2012). Analytes including GSH-Px, l-lactate (LAC), total glutathione (GSH-T), malondialdehyde (MDA), creatine kinase (CK), total leukocytes (WBC) and haematocrit (PCV) were determined.

All data was checked for normality of variance using the Shapiro-Wilks test in Proc Univariate & visual plotting in SAS 9.3. Many data sets were found not to have normal distributions and in each case power transformations or the natural logarithm were used. P-values stated here represent the transformed data comparisons, but lsmeans show values of the non-transformed data; for biological reference purposes. The effects of treatment, week, exercise period, sequence of treatment and all relevant interactions were analysed using ANOVA and repeated measures analysis in Proc Mixed (SAS Inst. Inc., Cary, NC). Pre-exercise values on each sampling week were also used as a covariate in the model. All differences were considered significant at $P<0.05$, with trends considered at $P<0.10$.

Results and discussion

All horses remained clinically healthy and sound throughout the trial. There was no difference due to the dietary treatment ($P>0.05$) for MDA, LAC, GSH-T, red blood cells (RBC), WBC and PCV overall throughout the training programme. The supplement had an overall treatment effect on GSH-Px ($P<0.05$) and CK ($P<0.01$). GSH-Px decreased in the CON group at the end of the blood sampling period following exercise in week 7 ($P<0.05$) (Figure 1).

Overall serum CK levels were lower in horses fed the supplement (treatment effect; $P<0.01$). The TRT group showed lower levels of CK throughout the training programme (treatment × week effect; $P<0.01$) (Figure 2), with the largest effect found in week 4 (CON = 208.8 ± 22.3, TRT = 134.97 ± 22.2 U/l) ($P<0.05$).

The TRT group's plasma CK levels remained significantly lower 24 hours post-exercise in this week ($P=0.0005$), whereas the CON group's CK levels were significantly elevated at this point (Figure 3). GSH-T levels showed a difference in week 7 only ($P=0.01$), with the CON group (25.6705 ± 0.88 uM) significantly higher than the TRT group (23.0762 ± 0.88 uM).

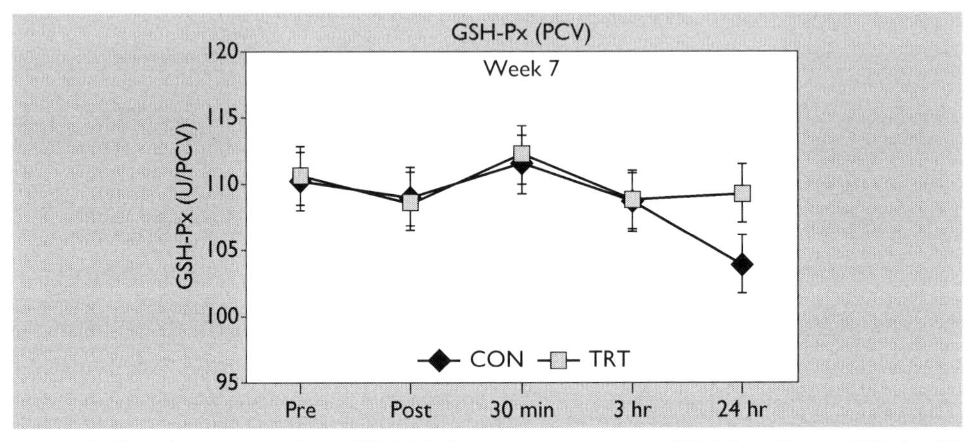

*Figure 1. Glutathione peroxidase (GSH-Px) for treatment groups CON (n=10) and TRT (n=10) before and after a sub-maximal exercise protocol, in week 7 of a training regime. * Significant differences between treatment groups at indicated time-point (P<0.05).*

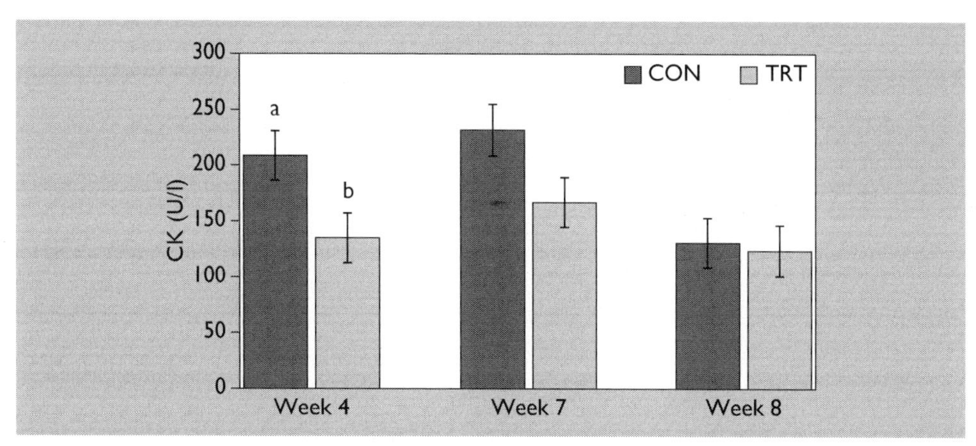

Figure 2. Creatine kinase (CK) activity of treatment groups CON (non-supplemented) and TRT (supplemented) throughout a training regime (weeks 4, 7 and 8). Different subscripts denote significant treatment effect within sampling weeks (P<0.01).

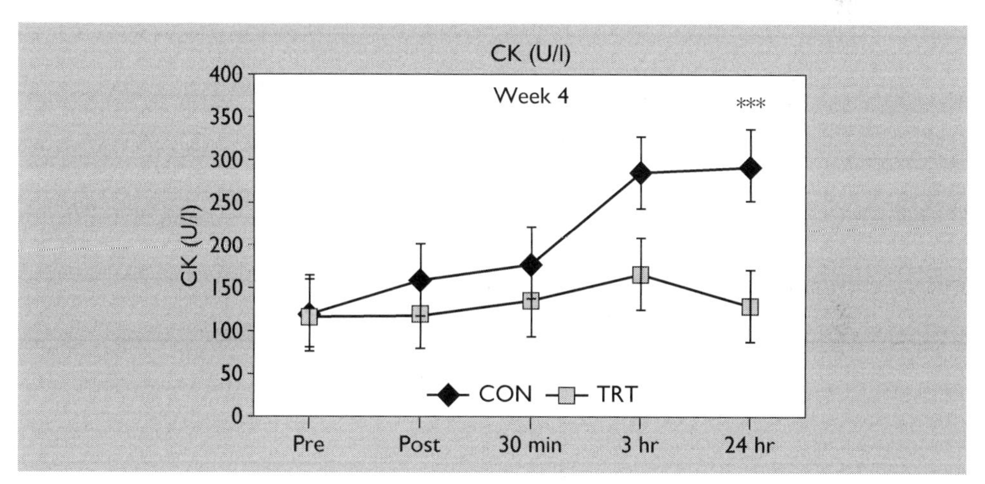

*Figure 3. Creatine kinase (CK) activity for treatment groups CON (n=10) and TRT (n=10) before and after a sub-maximal exercise protocol, in week 4 of a training regime. *** Significant differences between treatment groups at indicated time-points (P<0.001).*

Conclusion

The supplement used resulted in an increase in circulating enzymatic antioxidants in RBC GSH-Px concentrations. This increase may be of marked biological significance as it is this enzyme that is needed as a catalyst for utilizing GSH-T to scavenge ROS. Training or physical conditioning has been shown to reduce muscle cell leakage post-exercise especially at submaximal intensity even though there is a greater occurrence of exertional rhabdomyolysis at lower intensities (Siciliano *et al.*, 1995). It has been suggested that this increased capacity of cell membranes after conditioning is due to the strengthening of cell membranes and muscle fibres (Urso and Clarkson, 2003). It may be interesting as part of further research to investigate the effect this treatment will have in horses with a history of clinical exertional rhabdomyolysis and in horses trained at higher levels of intensity or durations of cardio vascular exertion. In this study we observed a reduction of almost 14% in CK levels in the supplemented group throughout the experiment. Other studies with single doses of antioxidant administrations of ascorbate (White *et al.*, 2001) and vitamin E (Siciliano *et al.*, 1997) were unable to show preventative post-exercise increases in plasma CK levels. The observation that the maximum effect on CK levels was at the beginning of the training programme (week 4) agrees with other studies (Freestone *et al.*, 1989; Siciliano *et al.*, 1995), which demonstrate that horses with lower basal antioxidant levels and/or fitness levels may be more prone to the negative effects of free radical damage in muscle cells. Thus pre-training or early training supplementation of this combination of natural exogenous ingredients will have maximal beneficial effects.

Acknowledgements

This research was sponsored by Connolly's Red Mills, Goresbridge, Ireland and Devenish Nutrition, Belfast, Northern Ireland.

References

Avellini, L., Chiaradia, E. and Gaiti, A., 1999. Effect of exercise training, selenium and vitamin E on some free radical scavengers in horses (*Equus caballus*). Comparative Biochemistry and Physiology B-Biochemistry & Molecular Biology 123: 147-154.

Freestone, J.F., Kamerling, S.G., Church, G., Bagwell, C. and Hamra, J., 1989. Exercise induced changes in creatine kinase and aspartate aminotransferase activities in the horse: effects of conditioning, exercise tests and acepromazine. Journal of Equine Veterinary Science 9: 275-280.

Lamprecht, E.D. and Williams, C.A., 2012. Biomarkers of antioxidant status, inflammation, and cartilage metabolism are affected by acute intense exercise but not superoxide dismutase supplementation in horses. Oxidative Medicine and Cellular Longevity 2012: 15.

Siciliano, P.D., Lawrence, L.M., Danielsen, K., Powell, D.M. and Thompson, K.N., 1995. Effect of conditioning and exercise type on serum creatine kinase and aspartate aminotransferase activity. Equine Vet J 27: 243-247.

Siciliano, P.D., Parker, A.L. and Lawrence, L.M., 1997. Effect of dietary vitamin E supplementation on the integrity of skeletal muscle in exercised horses. J Anim Sci 75: 1553-1560.

Urso, M.L. and Clarkson, P.M., 2003. Oxidative stress, exercise, and antioxidant supplementation. Toxicology 189: 41-54.

White, A., Estrada, M., Walker, K., Wisnia, P., Filgueira, G., Valdés, F., Araneda, O., Behn, C. and Martínez, R., 2001. Role of exercise and ascorbate on plasma antioxidant capacity in thoroughbred race horses. Comparative Biochemistry and Physiology Part A: Molecular & Integrative Physiology 128: 99-104.

Williams, C.A. and Carlucci, S.A., 2006. Oral vitamin E supplementation on oxidative stress, vitamin and antioxidant status in intensely exercised horses. Equine Vet J Suppl: 617-621.

M/L-ratio in long term intensive exercise training in Thoroughbreds used for racing and riding

G. Li, P. Lee, Y. Abe, N. Mori, I. Yamamoto and T. Arai
Department of Veterinary Science, School of Veterinary Medicine, Nippon Veterinary and Life Science University, 1-7-1 Kyonancho, Musashino, Tokyo 180-8602, Japan; ligebin@hotmail.com

Take home message

The sustained intensive training exercise regimen appears to result in increased energy metabolism efficiency in Thoroughbreds used for racing as opposed to Thoroughbreds used for riding, as evidenced by a higher plasma M/L ratio.

Introduction

Endurance training in horses can result in exercise-induced mitochondrial functional changes, such as marked increases in muscle mitochondrial respiration, although the adaptations appear to be muscle group specific (Votion *et al.*, 2010). Increased enzyme activity within the malate-aspartate shuttle appears to produce efficient energy metabolism in animal tissues (Arai *et al.*, 1998). In particular, malate dehydrogenase (MDH) is involved in gluconeogenesis and lipogenesis, playing a crucial role in the malate-aspartate shuttle (Setoyama *et al.*, 1988), transporting cytosolic NADH into mitochondria followed by oxidative ATP production (Hedeskov *et al.*, 1987). Alternately, lactate dehydrogenase (LDH) converts pyruvate to lactate consuming cytosolic NADH. Since cystosolic LDH activity is considered to be relatively stable under various metabolic conditions, cytosolic MDH/LDH (M/L) ratio can be a useful indicator for energy usage, and an increasing M/L ratio would reflect a heightened level of energy metabolism, including more ATP production in various animal tissues (Washizu *et al.*, 2001).

As a result of regular high intensity exercise training, race horses demonstrate significantly increased MDH activity levels when compared against riding horses (Arai *et al.*, 2002). The increase in MDH activity may be attributed to the fact that race horses have a more efficient energy producing system, especially in muscle, in order to maintain a high performance level for racing. Previous studies have advocated using M/L ratio of peripheral blood leucocytes (PBL) as an indicator of energy metabolism of Thoroughbred race horses (Arai *et al.*, 2002, 2001; Hosoya *et al.*, 2004). However, the use of PBL, as a cell source, for determining M/L ratio appears to be inconsistent, since M/L ratio was significantly higher for race horses as compared to riding horses in one study (Arai *et al.*, 2002), while it was not for another (Arai *et al.*, 2001), in spite of the fact that race horse MDH activity was higher than riding horses in both studies. The activity of PBL malate-aspartate shuttle enzymes may not directly reflect the ATP consumption rate by skeletal muscle, but instead is considered to be an indicator of the energy metabolism of the whole body in horses (Arai *et al.*, 2003). As such, the use of plasma instead of PBL may be more appropriate to determine M/L ratio.

Therefore, the aim of this study was to compare MDH, LDH activities, and M/L ratio between PBL and plasma of Thoroughbred race horses, as compared to that of Thoroughbred riding horses.

Materials and methods

All horses used in the study were Thoroughbreds, and were diagnosed by a veterinarian to be healthy and not pregnant in the case of mares. Five race horses (2 female and 3 male, 3-7 years old) were kept and trained at the Saitama Prefectural Urawa Horse racing Association`s Noda Training Center in Saitama, Japan. Each race horse usually exercised for 9 out of every 10 days, with the average 9 day workout regime consisting of: 3 days of fast galloping (13 to 18 m/s for 1000-1,200 m), and 6 days of slow work (6 to 8 m/s for 1,500-2,000 m), including warm-up and cool down for 2 h from 5:00 to 7:00 am. Five riding horses (6 to 22 years old, 1 female, 1 male and 3 geldings) were kept by the Saitama Riding Club Association in the same training center. Each riding horse was exercised by walking (2 to 3 m/s for 5 to 10 min) and trotting (4 to 6 m/s for 15 to 20 min) for 6 days on a weekly basis, resting on Sundays, over a 10 week period. All horses (race and riding) were maintained on grass supplemented with good-quality hay and concentrate. Blood was withdrawn from the jugular vein of resting horses into heparinized tubes, between 12:00 and 14:00 pm (~4 h post-prandial). Plasma was recovered by centrifugation at 3,500 rpm for 10 min at 4 °C and stored at -25 °C until subsequent use. Leucocytes were isolated by gradient centrifugation with LSM lymphocyte separation isolating solution (MP Biochemicals LLC,. Solon, OH, USA) following the manufacturer`s instructions. Cytosolic fractions of leucocytes were prepared and isolated according to the method previously described (Washizu *et al.* 1998). The activities of MDH and LDH in either the cytosolic fraction of leucocytes or plasma were measured by previously reported methods (LDH – Kaloustian *et al.*, 1969 and MDH – Bergmeyer and Brent, 1974). Protein concentration was determined by the Bradford (1976) method. The cytosolic M/L ratio was calculated as MDH specific activity divided by LDH specific activity.

Results

MDH, LDH, M/L ratio comparison between plasma and PBL in race and riding horses are presented in Table 1. Using PBL enzyme activities, MDH activity in race horses was significantly higher than that of riding horses. Alternately, when plasma was used instead, both MDH and LDH activities were significantly higher in race horses

Table 1. Comparison of MDH, LDH activities, and M/L Ratio between PBL and serum in race and riding horses. Values are presented as median with (range).

		Race horses (n=5)	Riding horses (n=5)
Cytosolic fraction of leukocytes	MDH (U/L)	393.00* (307.88-425.63)	248.58 (235.33-265.62)
	LDH (U/L)	769.96 (553.79-983.23)	622.38 (329.21-778.99)
	M/L ratio	0.51 (0.31-0.74)	0.41 (0.31-0.71)
Plasma	MDH(U/L)	433.88* (322.12-536.37)	112.60 (80.86-168.11)
	LDH (U/L)	193.01* (169.39-279.48)	111.21 (80.66-162.77)
	M/L ratio	2.04*,** (1.62-3.17)	1.00** (0.87-1.40)

* Denotes significant difference as compared to riding horses (Mann Whitney U-test, $P < 0.05$).

** Denotes significant difference as compared to PBL (Mann Whitney U-test, $P < 0.05$).

as compared to riding horses. These differences led to a significant increase in M/L ratio in race horses, which was twice that of riding horses (2.04 versus 1.0).

Discussion and conclusion

A higher M/L ratio may reflect elevated energy metabolism, including more ATP production, in some tissues such as muscle and liver. The use of plasma instead of PBL may be more appropriate to determine M/L ratio for several reasons. First, the isoenzyme pattern of LDH in horses differs between that of plasma and peripheral leucocytes, with LDH-1, -2, and -3 being dominant in plasma (Arai *et al.*, 2003; Hatzipanagiotou *et al.*, 1991); whereas LDH-3 and -4 are dominant in horse leucocytes (Arai *et al.*, 2003) suggesting a possible difference in LDH tissue source representation. These enzymes usually display different kinetic parameters (e.g. different KM values), or different regulatory properties. As such, LDH activity in serum may encompass more of the whole body as opposed to that exhibited by peripheral leucocytes. Secondly, because leucocytes are also involved in immune function and host defence against infectious diseases and foreign materials, any alteration in immune state may have an effect on energy metabolism, and in turn affect MDH activity levels.

This study has a number of limitations however. First, the small number of horses in each group ($n=5$) results in low statistical power, hence results and conclusions need to be interpreted with care. Second, riding horses used in our study were significantly older than the horses used for racing. Aging may have an impact on energy consumption, although higher MDH activities in skeletal muscle of older men undergoing endurance training have been observed suggesting that age may not be that influential (Suominen *et al.*, 1975).

In conclusion, an increase in plasma M/L ratio can reflect heightened energy metabolism in the liver and skeletal muscle of horses adapted to continuous intensive exercise.

References

Arai, T., Hosoya, M., Nakamura, M, Magoori, E., Uematsu, Y. and Sako, T., 2002. Cytosolic ratio of malate dehyrogenase/lactate dehydrogenase activity in peripheral leucocytes of race horses with training. Research in Veterinary Science 72: 241-244.

Arai, T., Inoue A, Uematsu, Y., Sako, T. and Kimura, N., 2003. Activities of enzymes in the malate-aspartate shuttle and the isoenzyme pattern of lactate dehydrogenase in plasma and peripheral leucocytes of lactating Holstein cows and riding horses. Research in Veterinary Science 75: 15-19.

Arai, T., Machida, T., Sasaki, M. and Oki, Y., 1998. Hepatic enzyme activities and plasma insulin concentrations in diabetic herbivorous voles. Veterinary Research Communications 13: 421-426.

Arai, T., Takahashi, M., Araki, K. and Washizu, T., 2001. Activities of enzymes related to the malate-aspartate shuttle in the blood cells of thoroughbred horses undergoing training exercise. Veterinary Research Communications 25: 577-583.

Bergmeyer, H.U. and Brent, E., 1974. Malate dehydrogenase UV assay. In: Bergmeyer, H.U. (ed.), Methods of enzymatic analysis, vol. 2. Verlag ChemieWeinheim Academic Press, New York, NY, USA, pp. 613-617.

Bradford, M.M., 1976. Rapid and sensitive method for the quantitation of microgram quantities of protein utilizing the principle of protein-dye binding. Analytical Biochemistry 72: 248-254.

Hatzipanagiotou, A., Lindner, A. and Sommer, H., 1991. LDH and CK isoenzyme patterns in the blood plasma of horses with elevated CK, LDH and AST activities. Deutsche Tierärztliche Wochenschrift 98: 284-286.

Hedeskov, J., Capito, K. and Thams, P., 1987. Cytosolic ratios of free [NADPH]/[$NADP^+$] and [NADH]/[NAD^+] in mouse pancreatic islets, and nutrient-induced insulin secretion. Biochemical Journal 241: 161-167.

Hosoya, M., Inoue, A., Kimura, N., Arai, T., 2004. Enzyme activities in some types of peripheral leukocytes of thoroughbred race horses before and after the races. Research in Veterinary Science 77:101-104.

Kaloustian, H.D., Stolzenbach, F.E., Everse, J., Kaplan, N.O., 1969. Lactate dehydrogenase of lobster (*Hornarus americanus*) tail muscle I. Physical and chemical properties. The Journal of Biological Chemistry 244:2891-2901.

Setoyama, C., Joh, T., Tsuzuki, T. and Shimada, K., 1988. Structural organization of the mouse cytosolic malate dehydrogenasegene: comparison with that of the mouse mitochondrial malate de hydrogenase gene. Journal of Molecular Biology 202: 355-364.

Suominen, H. and Heikkinen, E., 1975. Enzyme activities in muscle and connective tissue of M. vastus lateralis in habitually training and sedentary 33 to 70-year-old men. European Journal of Applied Physiology and occupational physiology 34: 249-254.

Votion, D.M., Fraipont, A., Goachet, A.G., Robert, C., van Erck, E., Amory, H., Ceusters, J., de la Rebière de Pouyade, G., Franck, T., Mouithys-Mickalad, A., Niesten, A. and Serteyn, D., 2010. Alterations in mitochondrial respiratory function in response to endurance training and endurance racing. Equine Veterinary Journal 42 Supplement 38: 268-274.

Washizu, T., Kuramoto, E., Abe, M., Sako, T. and Arai, T., 1998. A comparison of the activities of certain enzymes related to energy metabolism in leukocytes in dogs and cats. Veterinary Research Communications 22: 187-192.

Washizu, T., Takahashi, M., Azakami, D., Ikeda, M. and Arai, T., 2001. Activities of enzymes in the malate-aspartate shuttle in the peripheral leukocytes of dogs and cats. Veterinary Research Communications 25: 623-629.

Urinary parameters in horses supplemented with pulse dose of electrolytes

J.A. Martins, M.T. Ramos, A.C.T Miranda, L.A.G. Dimache, A.T. Silva, J.F. Azevedo, C.A.A. Oliveira, V.P. Silva, P. Trigo and F.Q. Almeida
Veterinary Institute, Universidade Federal Rural do Rio de Janeiro, BR 465, Km 07, Seropédica, RJ 23897-97, Brazil; falmeida@ufrrj.br

Take home message

Supplementation of high doses of electrolytes enhances water intake as well as urine production, changing drastically urine composition and enlarging its chloride and sodium concentration.

Introduction

Electrolytic supplementation in horses is a thoroughly used method that aims to attenuate dehydration and electrolytes losses, and helps rehydration in animals undergoing intense exercise or long trips (McCutcheon and Geor, 1996; Sampieri *et al.*, 2006). Most studies on electrolytes supplementation are performed on horses undergoing water stress, however studying mechanisms of regulation, as well as electrolytic interaction in horses during rest, can contribute for a better understanding of electrolytic supplementation. Thus, this study aimed to evaluate urinary parameters and water balance in horses at rest after pulse dose electrolytes supplementation.

Material and methods

This study was carried out at the Equine Health Laboratory at Universidade Federal Rural do Rio de Janeiro, Brazil. Experimental procedures were approved by the Ethics and Research Committee of UFRRJ, n.138/2011. A completely randomized 3 × 3 Latin Square design repeated in time was used with three animals and three treatments (electrolytic supplementation). Each experimental period comprised three days, totalling nine consecutive days, and electrolytes were supplied at day 1, day 4 and day 7. Treatments used were: Treatment 1 – control (without supplementation); Treatment 2 – supplementation with a medium dose of electrolytes composed by 0.25 g NaCl + 0.125 g KCl + 0.05 g CaCl + 0.025 g MgCl per kg of BW; Treatment 3 – supplementation with a high dose of electrolytes composed by 0.625 g of NaCl + 0.3125 g of KCl + 0.125 g of CaCl + 0.0625 g of MgCl per kg of BW, equivalent to 2.5 times the medium dose. The medium dose supplementation of electrolytes followed the recommendations of Sampieri *et al.* (2006), corresponding to electrolytic losses estimated for sweat production in one hour of intense exercise.

Two female and one male healthy adult crossbred horses, mean BW of 330 ± 38 kg, were used. The diet was provided in a forage:concentrate ratio of 70:30 composed by coastcross hay and concentrate, estimated intake of 2% BW, according to the NRC (2007) recommendations for horses at maintenance. All the animals received 116 mg/kg BW of mineral salt mixed to the concentrate.

To formulate the electrolytes supplementation pure salts were used: NaCl, KCl, MgCl and CaCl. Salts were weighted to adjust the dose to the animals' BW, diluted in two litres of deionized water, and delivered through nasogastric tube. One extra litre of deionized water was also delivered by the nasogastric tube with the purpose of rinsing the glass used for preparation and the tube itself, totalizing three litres. Animals in the control group received three litres of deionized water alone, delivered by nasogastric tube. On the day of the electrolytic supplementation horses were kept in their stalls and diet was supplied in two equal meals; at 4:00, four hours before the supplementation and the other half at 22:00, after the last sample collection. Samples were collected at the initial time of supplementation (zero) and at 2, 4, 6, 9 and 12 hours after supplementation.

Urine samples were collected through an urethral catheter and urine collector on the male, and by Foley catheter on the females. Catheters and collectors were prepared and placed three hours before the supplementation. Immediately after each sampling pH and electrical conductivity were measured. Total urine volume was measured with a beaker and weighted in a digital scale to allow calculation of density. Urine samples were stored in plastic containers and frozen for posterior analysis of sodium, potassium, chloride, calcium and magnesium. Urine output was measured during 12 hours after the treatments.

Feed analysis was performed on previously dried and ground samples, in a Willey mill (1-mm screen). Dry matter (DM) and mineral matter (MM) were determined according to AOAC (1995). Minerals analysis was performed by dry method. Water was analysed for sodium, potassium, chloride, calcium and magnesium, and performed directly and without dilution. Sodium and potassium analysis were performed on a Flame photometer. Calcium and magnesium analysis were performed in an Atomic absorption photometer. Chloride analysis was performed in spectrophotometer using commercial kits.

Data were submitted to ANOVA as a split-splot analysis and the mean values were compared by Tukey test at 5% probability using Statistics and Genetics Analysis System (SAEG).

Results

Water intake was influenced by the electrolytic supplementation at the times zero to 12 hours and zero to 24 hours (Table 1). There was no difference ($P>0.05$) on water intake from 12 to 24 hours after the electrolyte supplementation. Increase in water intake was observed from zero to 12 hours after the electrolyte supplementation and after that physiological responses could reestablish hydroelectrolytic balance.

Table 1. Water intake (ml/kg of BW) (means ± standard deviation) after electrolytic supplementation.

Time (hours)	Electrolytic supplementation[2]			CV%[1]
	Control	Medium	High	
0-12	10.6±7.9^{c}	32.5±6.5^{b}	67.2±14.7^{a}	26.8
12-24	28.2±6.0^{a}	24.4±8.4^{a}	24.8±4.4^{a}	22.4
0-24	38.7±10.5^{c}	56.9±5.3^{b}	92.0±14.5^{a}	17.7

[1] CV% = coefficient of variation.

[2] Mean values in line followed by different lower case letters differ by Tukey test ($P<0.05$).

Influence on water intake occurs in the first four hours after supplementation. Between 4 and 9 hours after supplementation, while water intake of horses from the medium dose treatment returned to values close to those of the control group, the high dose treatment horses remained elevated being the highest value 28.6 ± 22.8 ml/kg of BW.

The total excreted water was significantly influenced by the treatments, presenting, 19.9 ± 5.0; 30.7 ± 4.4 and 42.4 ± 10.5 ml of water/kg of BW for treatments control, medium dose and high dose, respectively. Those values correspond to the sum of water excreted in urine and faeces.

Animals receiving the high dose of electrolytes presented water retention 12 hours after supplementation, of 24.8 ± 10.2 ml/kg of BW. Treatment with medium dose did not differ when compared to control. Urine production, from time zero to 12 hours after supplementation increased significantly in high dose group, 27 ± 12.4 m/kg of BW, when compared to medium dose or control groups, 13 ± 5.1 and 7 ± 3.2, respectively, that did not differ (P>0.05) between them.

Urine density did not differ among treatments (P>0.05), but as a function of time (P<0.05), with a reduction at the fourth hour after the electrolyte supplementation, decreasing from 1.0671 to 1.0558 g/ml (Table 2). Urine pH did not differ as a function of treatment either

Table 2. Urine density and pH mean values of all treatments (means ± standard deviation)[1] after electrolytic supplementation.

Time (hours)	Density (g/ml)	pH
0	1.0671±0.008[a]	6.88±1.07[a]
2	1.0656±0.014[ab]	6.68±1.12[ab]
4	1.0522±0.009[c]	6.27±1.13[bc]
6	1.0531±0.014[c]	6.41±1.09[abc]
9	1.0540±0.014[c]	6.39±0.98[abc]
12	1.0558±0.013[bc]	6.05±0.88[c]
CV%[2]	1.0	8.2

[1] Mean values in columns followed by different lower case letters differ by Tukey test (P<0.05).

[2] CV% = coefficient of variation.

($P > 0.05$), however varied over time ($P < 0.05$), whereas the highest pH was observed before supplementation (time zero), 6.88, and lowest pH of 6.05 at 12 hours after supplementation.

Mean values of urine's electrical conductivity during 12 hours after supplementation differed ($P < 0.05$) as a function of treatments, with highest values observed in the medium dose group, of 43.24 ± 4.08 mS, and lowest values, of 34.94 ± 4.37 mS, in the control group, that did not differ from the high dose group.

The highest urinary sodium concentration during 12 hours after supplementation ($P < 0.05$) was observed in the high dose group (37.86 ± 14.05 mmol/l) and the lowest in the control group (21.38 ± 7.63 mmol/l), while the medium dose group (26.38 ± 24.16 mmol/l) did not differ from the two other treatments. Chloride urinary concentration during 12 hours after supplementation was higher ($P < 0.05$) in horses receiving the high and medium doses than control (182.77 ± 35.08 mmol/l, 206.21 ± 25.88 mmol/l and 144.65 ± 41.38 mmol/l respectively).

Urinary potassium and calcium concentration were not influenced by treatments ($P > 0.05$), but reduced with time. Mean value of potassium

Table 3. Mean urine values of magnesium (mmol/l) (means ± standard deviation) after electrolytic supplementation.

Time (hours)	**Electrolytic supplementation**[1]		
	Control	**Medium**	**High**
0	24.34±13.99^{Ba}	39.07±8.90^{Aba}	38.98±10.74^{Aa}
2	45.02±9.56^{Aabc}	29.95±14.70^{Aba}	21.18±6.97^{Bb}
4	17.47±9.26^{Abc}	16.17±5.25^{ABb}	9.30±7.78^{Bbc}
6	11.42±8.15^{Abc}	12.33±8.70^{ABb}	7.26±4.03^{Bc}
9	8.69±9.32^{Abc}	13.89±6.21^{Ab}	6.85±1.88^{Ac}
12	4.85±9.70^{Ac}	14.42±7.07^{Ab}	5.74±4.07^{Ac}

[1] Mean values in line followed by different capital letters differ by Tukey test (P<0.05). Mean values in columns followed by different lower case letters differ by Tukey test (P<0.05). CV (coefficient of variation) = 52.5%.

reduced from 146.52 mmol/l (time zero) to 97.77 mmol/l 12 hours after supplementation, and mean value of calcium reduced from 43.57 mmol/l (time zero) to 19.21 mmol/l 12 hours after supplementation. Therefore it is noticeable that increasing urine production enhances mineral excretion. There was effect of electrolyte supplementation and time after supplementation on urinary concentration of magnesium ($P < 0.05$), with higher values at time zero, decreasing to 12 hours after supplementation (Table 3).

Conclusions

Electrolytic supplementation enhanced the water intake, the water retention and the urine production in horses at rest. The supplementation influenced sodium and chloride concentration in urine also. Urine characteristics and the concentrations of Ca, K and Mg over time were significantly reduced.

References

Association of Official Analytical Chemists (AOAC), 1995. Official methods of analysis, 16th ed. AOAC International, Arlington, VA, USA.

McCutcheon, L.J. and Geor, R.J., 1996. Sweat fluid and ion losses in horses during training and competition in cool vs. hot ambient conditions: implications for ion supplementation. Equine Veterinary Journal Suppement 22: 54-62.

National Research Council (NRC), 2007. Nutrient requirements of horses. 6th ed. Washington, DC, USA.

Sampieri, F., Schott II, H. C., Hinchcliff, K. W., Geor, R. J. and Jose-Cunilleras, E., 2006. Effects of oral electrolyte supplementation on endurance horses competing in 80 km rides. Equine Veterinary Journal Supplement 36: 19-26.

The influence of boot design on exercise associated skin surface temperature covering tendons in horses

L. Sander[1], L. Hopegood[2] and A.D. Ellis[3]
[1]Hofgut Beutig, 04749 Ostrau, Germany; [2]Nottingham Trent University, School of Animal, Rural and Environmental Sciences, Brackenhurst, Southwell, Nottinghamshire NG25 0QF, United Kingdom; [3]UNEQUI, Research, Education and Innovation; Southwell, Nottinghamshire NG25 0DS, United Kingdom; lyn.hopegood@ntu.ac.uk

Take home message

Boots designed with perforations reduced tendon exposure to high temperatures in this study and thus may protect against tendon injury.

Introduction

The most common injuries in sports horses are related to the superficial digital flexor tendon (SDFT) and the deep digital flexor tendon of the distal limb (Murray *et al.*, 2006). In order to prevent mechanical injury to these structures boots are worn during competitions but the possible resultant increase in heat stress to these areas is unknown. Boots counteract any natural cooling mechanism by preventing heat dissipation. Boot materials and design vary and recently the focus on allowing air circulation has increased. Lining material used such as neoprene is known for its thermoregulatory properties (Bardy *et al.*, 2006) and may 'conserve' and lock in heat. Thermoplastic elastomers are also used for their softness and durability (Holden *et al.*, 2000). Combining these materials may provide thermal insulation thus heating the surface of the skin and the tendon beneath.

Release of stored energy in a tendon results in heat production in the SDFT to as much as 45 °C in horses on a treadmill (Wilson and Goodship, 1994). When tendons were exposed *in vitro* to 45 °C only 27%

of tenocytes survived, as blood supply in the tendon is insufficient to cool the limb (Yamasaki *et al.*, 2001). Temperatures of 46-48 °C over a period of 10 minutes resulted in a rapid change in matrix composition and decline of tendon fibroblast activity possibly resulting in cell death (Birch *et al.,* 1997). The loss of tendon cells is the main feature of tendonitis and the number of apoptic tenocytes in inflamed SDFTs is significantly higher than in normal tendons (Hosaka *et al.*, 2005). For that reason the tendon should be kept as cool as possible (Petrov *et al.*, 2003). These considerations have only recently been taken into consideration when designing horse boots through the addition of air perforations.

The aim of this study was to measure the effect of different types of boots on skin surface temperature covering the SDFT and heat dissipation temperature from those boots in a controlled study and during an applied field test.

Materials and methods

Temperature measurements

Designed originally for engineering purposes, infra-red thermography (IRT) is useful non-invasively and is an ideal tool to use to study limb and boot surface temperatures in this present study. The Raytek Raynger ST20 (Berlin, Germany; range of -32 to 535 °C) was used to measure temperatures. Measurements were taken approximately 5 cm from the limb.

Controlled study

Four sound German Warmblood horses (550 ± 50 kg bodyweight, 6-13 years old) were selected. Pre-test temperatures of their legs were taken before and after exercise to ensure there were no injuries or soundness issues around the tendons or boot areas. The Eskadron (Werther, Germany) cross country boot and the New Equine Wear Air flow (Cardigan, Wales, UK) boots were tested on all four limbs. The study consisted of two parts, a lungeing test and a ridden exercise test which took place over four days in a cross-over design. Each test was performed twice and horses wore one set of boots (e.g. Eskadron) on left limbs while wearing the other set (e.g. Air flow) on the opposite leg in a further cross-over design. Therefore, each leg was used as a separate unit with opposite leg as control treatment so that measures were taken simultaneously reducing any environmental effects. Measures were always taken in the same order to eliminate timing results. Horses were lunged for 15 minutes each containing walk (6 minutes), trot (8 minutes) and canter (1 minute) split in equal amounts between directions. After the exercise, temperatures were taken in three areas to assess heat dissipation with the boot still in place: just above the boot (top; 1), in the middle of the boot (middle; 2) and just below the boot (bottom; 3) on all four legs.

The ridden exercise test (same rider) was carried out in an arena with a sand surface and included 10 minutes warm up in walk, 5 minutes of trot in each direction and 2.5 minutes canter on each rein. Measurements of all four limbs were again taken.

Field test

The field test was carried out in October at the International Horse Trials at Aldon. Horses from two classes were used, namely the BE100 three day class with roads and tracks (n=61) and a CCI* (n=69) in short format. Twenty-one different types of boots were recorded at the event. For data analysis boots were pooled into three groups: a conventional boot design (closed all around the leg = conventional; n=93), boots with a design using holes, perforations or mesh design to allow for air to cool the leg (air cooled, n=24) and open fronted tendon boots (tendon boots; n=12). Temperatures were taken immediately after horses crossed the finish line of the cross country phase after the boot had been removed. Temperatures of the left front leg only of the horses were taken laterally mid-way between the carpus and the metacarpophalangeal joint on the SDFT.

Statistical analysis

Statistical analysis was carried out using IBM SPSS (v17.00). The significance level was set as $P<0.05$. Data were analysed for normal distribution and for the controlled study Univariate ANOVA was applied, testing for differences between boots and for effects and interactions between left and right, fore and hind, exercise and phases.

An ANOVA-Bonferroni was used to test for differences between boots during the field test and to test for effect of class.

Results

Controlled study

There were no effects according to left and right legs or phases. When all temperature areas (top, middle and bottom) were considered together there was no significant difference in heat dissipation between the two boots (Figure 1). There was a significant difference in heat dissipation in the middle area between exercises and between boots ($P<0.01$) (Table 1).

Field test

There was no significant difference in limb temperatures between the two eventing classes. There was a significantly lower temperature for tendon boots compared to conventional boots ($P<0.05$) and Air cooled boots compared to conventional boots ($P<0.001$). There was also a significantly lower temperature in Air cooled boots compared to tendon boots ($P<0.001$) (Table 2).

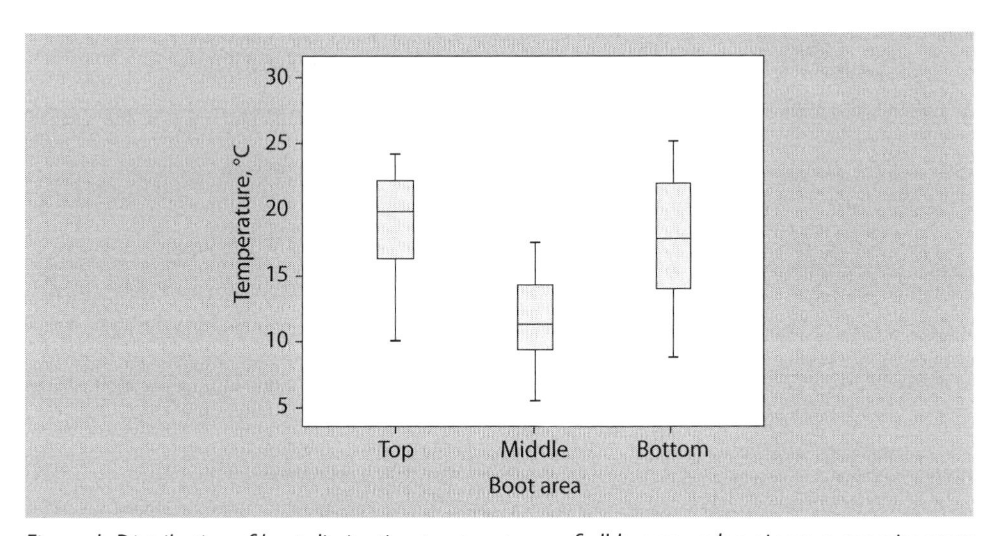

Figure 1. Distribution of heat dissipation temperatures of all horses undergoing two exercise tests and wearing two types of boot depending on area.

Table 1. Mean heat dissipation temperature from outer surface in the middle of the boot according to boots and exercise for 4 horses.

	Treatment	Temperature (°C)[1]	P-value[2]	n
Eskadron	Lunging	11.63±1.9	0.064, F=5.1	4
	Ridden	8.54±1.9		
Airflow	Lunging	15.46±2.0	0.074, F=4.7	4
	Ridden	12.00±2.9		
Boots[3]	Eskadron	10.08±2.4	0.005, F=11	8
	Airflow	13.73±3.0		
Exercise[4]	Lunging	13.54±2.7	0.009, F=9.6	8
	Ridden	10.27±3.0		

[1] Mean value ± standard deviation.

[2] Univariate Anova.

[3] ×2 exercises.

[4] ×2 boots.

Table 2. Mean, minimum and maximum temperatures of skin surface according to type of boot for 129 horses upon completion of the cross country phase of a one day event.

Boot Type	n	Mean[1]	Standard error	Min	Max
Conventional	93	32.33 ^{a}	±0.17	29.3	36.5
Air cooled	12	28.66 ^{b}	±0.32	25.6	32.6
Tendon boot	24	31.10 ^{c}	±0.47	28.9	33.4
No Boot[2]	2	21.70		21.2	22.2

[1] Anova, Bonferroni: superscripts ^{ab}, ^{bc} $P<0.001$; ^{ac} $P<0.05$.

[2] Not included in statistical analysis.

Discussion

Infra-red thermography was ideal for temperature measurements in the competition environment, as it could be used quickly and easily. It is, however, very important when using IRT to take into account air temperature and radiation heat related to strength of sunlight. The slightly unconventional application of different boots on opposing legs was used in the controlled study to help eliminate these influences. Good repeatability was shown with consistency between legs, justifying the use of only four horses. In the controlled study there was a significant difference between the boots ($P < 0.01$) in the middle of the boots only. These results showed that the Airflow boots allowed for greater heat dissipation by a mean of 3 °C.

As the temperature of the middle of the boots during lungeing was higher than during riding, lungeing appeared more strenuous (exercise duration and paces were kept similar). This may reflect the biomechanical use of the limb on a circle, resulting in a greater workload (Van Oldruitenborgh-Oosterbaan *et al.*, 1991).

During the field study the insulating effect of boots was shown as limb temperatures of the two horses competing without boots were approximately 22 °C (BE100) which were considerably lower than those wearing boots (total mean 30.7 °C). In light of tendon injuries being one of the most common injuries in sports horses (Murray *et al.*, 2006) it is interesting to note that 81% (105 out of 129) of riders recorded at this event still used the conventional or back closed tendon boots.

The maximum skin surface temperatures in the present study were measured at 36.5 °C for conventional boots. With the average tendon core being 5.4 °C warmer than the skin temperature (Wilson and Goodship, 1994) potentially damaging temperatures of 41.9 °C were reached with these boots during the field study. Birch *et al.* (1997) reported that a tendon temperature of 39 °C leads to a 4% decrease of tendon fibroblast viability compared to 37 °C. Therefore, there is considerable cause for concern as to the viability of tendon fibroblasts when competing in certain boots. Maximum temperatures reached by air cooled boots were less alarming.

Conclusion

The type of boot worn influenced the heat produced under the boot during exercise. Designs to cool the horse's leg by introduction of perforations or holes to allow airflow showed higher temperature dissipation in the middle of the boot and lower skin surface temperature than closed conventional boots. Boots should be designed to minimise tendon exposure to high temperatures and thus protect against tendon injury and potential welfare implications.

Acknowledgements

Thanks go to the whole team at Aldon Horse Trials for accommodating the study. Further thanks go to all the riders that participated.

References

Bardy, E., Mollendorf, J. and Pendergast, D., 2006. A comparison of the thermal resistance of a foam neoprene wetsuit to a wetsuit fabricated from aerogel-syntactic foam hybrid insulation. Journal of Physics D: Applied Physics 39: 4068-4076.

Birch, H.L., Wilson, A.M. and Goodship, A.E., 1997. The effect of exercise induced hyperthermia on tendon cell survival. Journal of Experimental Biology 200: 1703-1708.

Holden, G., Kricheldorf, H.R. and Quirk, R.P., 2000. Thermoplastic Elastomers. 3rd ed. Hanser, OH, USA.

Hosaka Y., Teraoka H., Yamamoto E., Ueda, H. and Takehana K., 2005. Mechanism of cell death in inflamed superficial digital flexor tendon in the horse. Journal of Comparative Pathology 132: 51-58.

Murray, R.C., Dyson, S.J., Tranquille, C. and Adams, V., 2006. Association of type of sport and performance level with anatomical site of orthopaedic injury diagnosis. Equine Veterinary Journal 38: 411-416.

Petrov, R., MacDonald, M.H., Tesch, A.M. and Van Hoogmoed, L.M., 2003. Influence of topic applied cold treatment on core temperature and cell viability in equine superficial digital flexor tendons. American Journal of Veterinary Research 64: 835-844.

Van Oldruitenborgh-Oosterbaan, M.M.S., Wensing, T.H., Barnefeld, A. and Breukink, H.J., 1991. Work-load in the horse during vaulting competition. In: Persson S.G.B., Lindholm A., Jeffcott L.B. (eds.) Equine Exercise Physiology 3, ICEEP Publications Davis, California, USA, pp. 331-336.

Wilson, A.M. and Goodship, A.E., 1994. Exercise-induced hyperthermia as a possible mechanism for tendon degeneration. Journal of Biomechanics 27: 899-905.

Yamasaki, H., Goto, M., Yoshihara, T., Sekigushi, M., Konno, K., Momoi, Y. and Iwasaki, T., 2001. Exercise-induced superficial digital flexor tendon hyperthermia and the effect of cooling sheets on thoroughbreds. Journal of Equine Science 12: 85-91.

Free fatty acid and antioxidant profiles in athletic horses: relationship to clinical status and performance

E. van Erck and J. Dauvillier
Equine Sports Medicine Practice, 83 Avenue Beau Séjour, 1410 Waterloo, Belgium; info@esmp.be

Take home message

Plasma free fatty acid (FFA) and antioxidant profiles vary according to age, type of discipline and in some circumstances to clinical status in working equine athletes. Standardization of sampling is recommended to improve the reliability of results. Some omega 6 and omega 3 FFA, glutathion peroxidase (GPx) and vitamin E are significantly correlated and appear as the parameters of most interest in equine sports medicine. Supplementation of fat and antioxidants should be carefully assessed and closely adapted to the horse's type and level of activity.

Introduction

Horses are naturally athletic animals that are able to reach exceptionally high levels of oxygen consumption during exercise. Fat metabolism represents an important source of energy in athletes performing exercise of moderate to low intensity exercise. Oil is routinely added to equine diets and is perceived as potentially beneficial for performance. An elevation of plasma free fatty acid (FFA) concentration prior to exercise has been previously reported to increase fat utilisation in horses during low intensity exercise (Orme *et al.*, 1995). Increased fat dietary content is advocated to increase the energetic density of a diet or to reduce carbohydrate intake in certain pathological circumstances. It has also been suggested that in horses, free fatty acids could potentially be used as indices of energy status and health (Gordon *et al.*, 2009).

However, in humans high fat intake is known to promote oxidative stress. Plasma fatty acid concentrations were found to be positively correlated with pro-inflammatory and pro-oxidative markers. Although the underlying mechanism is uncertain, this effect may be a direct effect of increased free radical generation during fat metabolism or an indirect effect of increased metabolic rate resulting from increased energy intake (Loft *et al.*, 1998).

The aim of this study was to evaluate the FFA and the anti-oxidant profiles in working horses practising different disciplines and correlate these indices to clinical status and performance.

Material and methods

The studied population included 103 horses in training referred for a seasonal athletic check-up or poor performance. Age, gender, breed, equestrian discipline and level as well as medical history were recorded. The horses underwent a clinical examination, a standardised exercise test and a blood sample. In cases referred for poor performance, further ancillary exams were undertaken to establish a diagnosis (resting or exercising endoscopy, echocardiography, etc.).

A clinical score (/3) was attributed according to the following criteria:
- Score 1. Healthy status and good performance.
- Score 2. Diagnosis of a disease compatible with the pursuit of training but causing decreased performances.
- Score 3. Diagnosis of a disease incompatible with the normal pursuit of training and causing exercise intolerance.

Performance evaluation was based on owner perception, outcome of the standardised exercise test and performance records.

The blood sample was taken in the morning prior to exercise. It included routine haematology and biochemistry parameters. The measured antioxidant markers were gluthation peroxidase (GPx), superoxide dismuthase (SOD), vitamin E (VitE), vitamin A (VitA), Coenzyme Q10 (CoQ10), selenium (Se), Zinc (Zn), Copper (Cu). The measured FFA were:
- the saturated FFA: myristic, palmitic, stearic and pentadecylic acids;

- the monounsaturated FFA: palmitoleic, cis-vaccenic, oleic and gadoleic acids;
- the trans FFA: trans-vaccenic and elaïdic acid;
- the omega 6 (n-6) FFA: linoleic, gammalinolenic, dihomogamma-linolenic (DGLA), arachidonic (AA) and docosapentanoeic acids;
- the omega 3 (n-3) FFA: alphalinolenic (LN), eicosapentaenoeic (EPA), docosahexaenoic (DHA) acids;
- the global n-6/n-3 ratio, AA/EPA and LN/DGLA ratios.

A multivariate analysis of variance for FFA and antioxidant markers was done using the GLM procedure on SAS. No interaction terms were included in the models. Chi-square tests and student t-test were used to analyse separately the potential association across all surveyed effects (age, gender discipline, etc.). Pearson's correlation was used to study the relationship between FFA and anti-oxidant markers.

Results

Global FFA and antioxidant parameters are summarized in Tables 1 and 2, respectively. Some FFA and antioxidant parameters show strong inter-individual variations. Some variability can be attributed to age and equestrian discipline.

The equestrian disciplines represented were 54% showjumping, 7% eventing, 6% dressage, 13% endurance, 17% standardbred race, 4% active pleasure. Both FFA and anti-oxidant profiles varied according to discipline, namely AA/EPA being highest in dressage horses and lowest in endurance horses and standardbred racehorses had the lowest values in saturated FFA and highest values in VitE and Se.

Gender did not have a significant influence on any of the measured parameters; however FFA profiles significantly differed with age, with younger horses having higher plasmatic values for almost all FFA. The LNA, GLNA and n-6/n-3 ratio were positively correlated to VitE. The n-6/n-3, AA/EPA ratios and DHA were positively correlated to GPx, VitE and Se. The EPA and LN as well as LN/DGLA were negatively correlated to GPx.

Regarding the clinical status, 48.4% of horses had a clinical score of 3, 19.3% a score of 2 and 30.3% a score of 1.

Table 1. Mean values and standard deviation (SD) of plasmatic free fatty acids in 103 athletic horses.

Fatty acid	Mean (µmol/l)	SD
Myristic acid	8.1	9.1
Palmitic acid	438.7	131.7
Stearic acid	576.7	160.4
Pentadecylic acid	5.0	2.2
Palmitoleic acid	11.1	11.1
Cis-vaccenic acid	21.8	6.7
Oleic acid	212.2	81.0
Gadoleic acid	8.9	3.3
Trans-vaccenic acid	2.3	1.8
Elaïdic acid	2.2	2.2
Linoleic acid	905.9	222.2
Gammalinolenic acid	3.4	5.1
Dihomogammalinolenic acid	16.6	5.9
Arachidonic acid	37.4	11.1
Docosapentanoeic acid	3.7	12.5
Alphalinolenic acid	38.4	37.2
Eicosapentaenoeic acid	4.8	7.1
Docosahexaenoic acid	3.1	1.6
n-6/n-3 ratio	28.8	14.9
AA/EPA[1]	11.5	6.1
LN/DGLA[1]	83.8	175.7

[1] AA/EPA: arachidonic acid/eicosapentaenoeic acid ratio; LN/DGLA: alphalinolenic acid/dihomogammalinolenic acid ratio.

The DHA was positively correlated with GPx and performance levels ($P<0.01$). Results failed to demonstrate a significant correlation between any of the FFA or antioxidant markers and general clinical status however it appeared that horses diagnosed with respiratory diseases had higher LNA levels.

Discussion and conclusions

The FFA and antioxidant profiles are highly variable in horses according to age and equestrian discipline. These variations can be due to variations in diet, time of feeding as well as differences in

Table 2. Mean values and standard deviation (SD) of antioxydants in 103 athletic horses.

Antioxydant	Mean (μmol/l)	SD
GPx[1]	721.1	45.7
SOD[1]	911.4	290.6
Vitamin E	5.2	1.8
Vitamin A	22.8	10.3
Coenzyme Q10	116.3	43.3
Selenium	164.5	40.9
Zinc	73.6	20.3
Copper	108.5	24.5

[1] GPx: gluthation peroxydase; SOD: superoxide dismuthase.

physical activity, training status and competitive level. Standardization of sampling would be recommended to improve the reliability of results as some FFA show strong circadian changes (Orme *et al.*, 1995). Plasma FFA are known to display higher variability than erythrocytic FFA. The measurement of the latter parameter may be more reliable, although it represents structural implementation of FFA and cannot reflect more immediate changes in FFA metabolism.

This study shows that, in the population considered, endurance horses and showjumpers competing at high-level could have benefited from diets enriched in n-3 FFA. Although such observations were made for several horses, diet was not systematically recorded and further research should be conducted to evaluate this point. Because of the negative correlation with n-3 FFA, anti-oxidant supplementation might be recommended in fat-enriched diets to ensure acceptable levels of protective GPx and VitE. More refined analysis should also be undertaken in specific horse populations, and interpretation of individual results should be made taking into account the equestrian discipline and level. Furthermore DHA, an exogenous n-6 FFA, is correlated to performance. It is unclear whether this is linked to specific diets in horses competing at higher level or if it represents an adaptation of the energy metabolism leading to improved performances. In any event, an evaluation of individual diet composition should be undertaken to reliably interpret plasmatic FFA profiles.

The production of reactive oxygen species is boosted by physical exercise and training (Hargreaves *et al.*, 2002; Kirschvink *et al.*, 2002); in these circumstances; the risk of damage to cells and tissues is increased (Clarkson and Thompson, 2000). In man, exercise-induced oxidative stress contributes to the acceleration of muscle fatigue and muscle fibre damage (Sen and Packer, 2000). The level of oxidative stress has been correlated to the intensity and duration of exercise (De Moffarts *et al.*, 2005; Gondim *et al.*, 2009; Williams *et al.* 2005) as well as to performance (Gondim *et al.*, 2009). In this study, the good performers had the highest levels of GPx and vitamin E. This can be linked to diet but also to training-induced adaptations.

It appears that FFA and antioxidant profile analysis can be useful to assess the quality of the horse's diet and assess if the diet meets the specific individual requirements. It could also be useful to monitor the variations in the horse's health status during a competitive season.

References

Clarkson, P.M. and Thompson, H.S., 2000. Antioxidants: what role do they play in physical activity and health? American Journal of Clinical Nutrition 72 Supplement 2: 637S-646.

De Moffarts, B., Kirschvink, N., Art, T., Pincemail, J. and Lekeux, P., 2005. Effect of oral antioxidant supplementation on blood antioxidant status in trained Thoroughbred horses. Veterinary Journal 169: 65-74.

Gondim, F.J., Zoppi, C.C., Dos Reis Silveira, L., Pereira-Da-Silva, L. and Vaz De Macedo, D., 2009. Possible relationship between performance and oxidative stress in endurance horses. Journal of Equine Veterinary Science 29: 206-212.

Gordon, M.E., Jerina, M.L., Raub, R.H., Davison, K.A., Young, Y.K. and Williamson, K.K., 2009. The effects of dietary manipulation and exercise on weight loss and related indices of health in horses. Comparative Exercise Physiology 6: 33-42.

Hargreaves, B.J., Kronfeld, D.S., Waldron, J.N., Lopes, M.A., Gay, L.S., Saker, K.E., Cooper, W.L., Sklan, D.J. and Harris P.A., 2002. Antioxidant Status And muscle cell leakage during endurance exercise. Equine Veterinary Journal 34: 116-121.

Kirschvink, N., Smith, N., Fievez, L., Bougnet, V., Art, T., Degand, G., Marlin, D., Roberts, C., Genicot, B., Lindsey, P. and Lekeux, P., 2002. Effect of chronic airway inflammation and exercise on pulmonary and systemic antioxidant status of healthy and heaves-affected horses. Equine Veterinary Journal 34: 563-571.

Loft, S., Thorling, E.B. and Poulsen, H.E., 1998. High fat diet induced oxidative DNA damage estimated by 8-oxo-7,8-dihydro-2-deoxyguanosine excretion in rats. Free Radical Research 29: 595-600.

Orme, C.E., Harris, R.C. and Marlin, D.J., 1995. Effect of elevated plasma FFA on fat utilisation during low intensity exercise. Equine veterinary Journal Supplement 18: 199-204.

Sen, C.K. and Packer, L., 2000. Thiol homeostasis and supplements in physical exercise. American Journal of Clinical Nutrition 72: 653S-669S.

Williams, C.A., Kronfeld, D.S., Hess, T.M., Saker, K.E., Waldron, J.E., Crandell, L.M. and Harris, P.A., 2005. Comparison of oxidative stress and antioxidant status in endurance horses in three 80-km races. Equine and Comparative Exercise Physiology 2: 153-157.

Related titles:

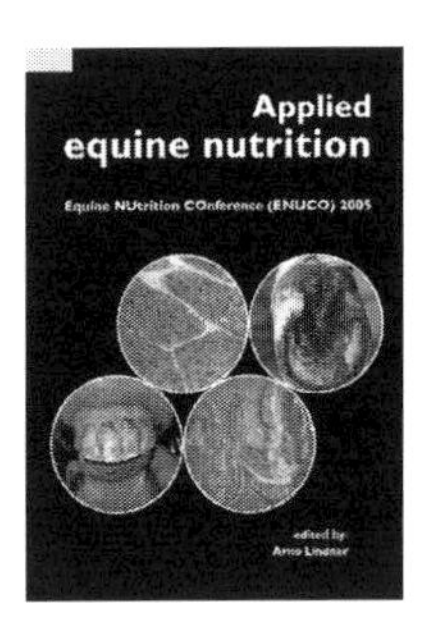

Applied equine nutrition
Equine NUtrition COnference (ENUCO) 2005
edited by: Arno Lindner
paperback ISBN 978-90-76998-85-5
e-book ISBN 978-90-8686-563-5
www.WageningenAcademic.com/ENUCO2005

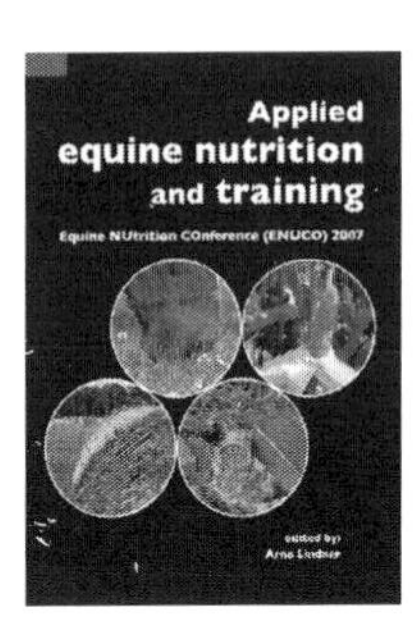

Applied equine nutrition and training
Equine NUtrition COnference (ENUCO) 2007
edited by: Arno Lindner
paperback ISBN 978-90-8686-040-1
e-book ISBN 978-90-8686-607-6
www.WageningenAcademic.com/ENUCO2007

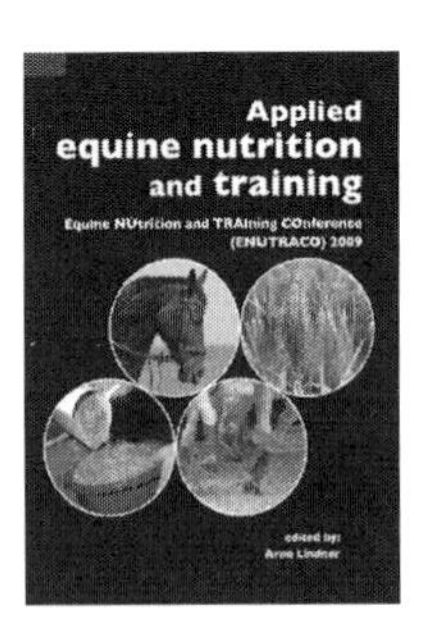

Applied equine nutrition and training
Equine NUtrition and TRAining COnference (ENUTRACO) 2009
edited by: Arno Lindner
paperback ISBN 978-90-8686-124-8
e-book ISBN 978-90-8686-669-4
www.WageningenAcademic.com/ENUTRACO2009

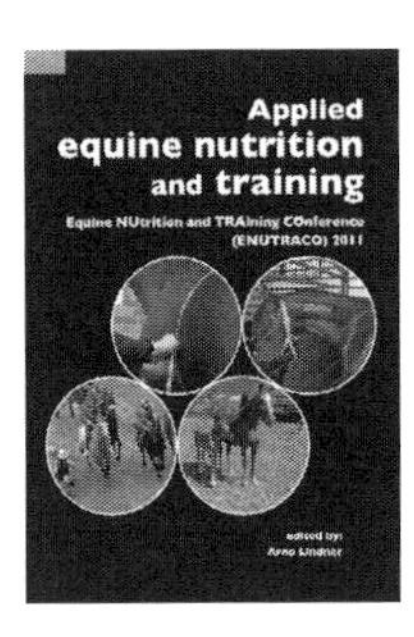

Applied equine nutrition and training
Equine NUtrition and TRAining COnference (ENUTRACO) 2011
edited by: Arno Lindner
paperback ISBN 978-90-8686-183-5
e-book ISBN 978-90-8686-740-0
www.WageningenAcademic.com/ENUTRACO2011

Printed in the United States
by Baker & Taylor Publisher Services